COPYCAT RESTAURANT FAVORITES

A Guide and Compilation of the Most-Loved, Healthy, and Easy Favorite Copycat Restaurant Recipes that you can Cook in the Comfort of Your Own Home

Melissa Pot

TABLE OF CONTENTS

Introduction

With a recession scare creeping across the economy and your budget likely getting a very tight squeeze, you're probably looking for some way to stretch it out and make it last. Do you believe that Copycat Recipes will help you recover any, perhaps a whole bunch of dollars in your budget?

It will certainly do that, and once you look at it, it's simple math. In making copycat recipes you'll not only save a lot on the expense of' eating out' but also on gas, and that's a huge bonus. Just to offer a quick example, and these are very conservative figures, if you eat out just twice a week and spend around $45 in the sum of each dinner out, that is $360 a month. Note, this doesn't even include the cost of driving to your favorite locations. Many people probably spend a lot more than eating out each month, depending on where you are going and how many people you are shopping for. Do you see how much money you can save by making these homemade meals?

The question you might ask is, how can you cook a dish or meal from scratch, with your own ingredients that will taste as good as what you can find at your favorite restaurant or eating establishment? It is easy when you can get your hands on a strong Copycat Recipes set or source.

These are reverse engineered recipes that were passed down from some of the original chefs who created the popular meals in the restaurants. It helps you to design and recreate recipes of previously hidden dishes for use and enjoyment in your home. So close, as a matter of fact, that you wouldn't be able to tell the difference between the one you cooked and the one from the restaurant!

So, by accessing Copycat Recipes, you can basically make your family super happy by serving their favorite meals whenever they want, and put a bunch of money back into your pocket every month by wiping out your monthly "eating out" budget!

If you are having a party, you can make a copycat restaurant recipe that will have your guests swearing you purchased it from the restaurant that made the dish famous. You can enjoy the attention your cooking will bring when you decide to make a copycat restaurant recipe for your next party or potluck dinner.

Just because you cook your own food doesn't mean it can't be as delicious as a five-star restaurant; all you need are a few simple tools. You don't have to be a master chef to cook like one, either. The equipment needed to prepare the recipes in this book are broken into appliances, cooking gadgets, cookware, and bakeware. You will also learn the terms and techniques needed to make a wonderful restaurant-quality meal.

The Essential Kitchen Gear

Appliances

These appliances will provide the greatest convenience and versatility in your kitchen:

- Electric mixer — A portable handheld mixer will do well for all of the recipes in this book.

- Blender — This kitchen helper cuts time instantly by blending, chopping, and puréeing foods.

- Deep fryer — A small Fry Daddy is the best at regulating the temperature of the cooking oil when deep frying meats or vegetables.

- George Foreman Indoor Grill — This is a great time saver in the kitchen when grilling any kind of meat, since both sides cook at once.

- Microwave oven — As ubiquitous as they are, you can rely on them for quick thawing and heating jobs in the kitchen.

Cooking Gadgets

A good cook knows that a good-quality set of knives can accomplish more in the kitchen than any electronic device. These are the knives that you will need:

- A chef's knife that has a broad, tapered shape, which can easily be rocked over ingredients.

- A bread knife, which has a serrated edge that makes it perfect for cutting through crusts.

- A paring knife has a short blade that is used for peeling, trimming, coring, and seeding vegetables.

Cooking in the kitchen can be fun, but it is a spot for potential accidents. There are some basic safety rules you should follow to make your cooking experience more enjoyable: The kitchen is not the place to go barefoot; it is important to understand your tools and how to handle them properly; read the instructions on how to use your appliances.

Other Tools

Other tools needed in food preparation include:

- Bottle opener

- Can opener

- Colander

- Cutting board

- Grater

- Long-handled forks, spoons, and spatulas

- Meat mallet

- Pizza cutter

- Rolling pin

- Set of measuring cups

- Set of measuring spoons

- Set of mixing bowls

Cookware

You'll also need the following pieces of cookware:

- Saucepans with lids (small, medium, and large)

- Stockpot (large enough to make soup for your family)

- Cast-iron skillet (for using in the oven)

- 12" nonstick skillet

Bakeware

Don't forget these necessary pieces of bakeware:

- Baking sheets

- Casserole dishes (small, medium, and large)

- Muffin pan

- Rectangular sheet cake pan

- Roasting pan with a rack

- Pizza pan

Stocking the Pantry

Cooking is much easier when you know what you've already got on hand and aren't running to the grocery store every time you want to fix a meal. Having a well-stocked pantry is a cook's secret weapon. Here is a list of basic ingredients that should be in your pantry. Of course, you can adjust items on the list to suit your family's likes and dislikes.

Herbs and Spices

If you've spent any time in the spice aisle at the supermarket lately, you know how expensive spices are. A little bottle will set you back a couple of bucks. Therefore, it is recommended that you buy seasoning blends. Some of the most common and widely used flavors are:

- Barbecue seasoning, which contains a variety of spices that are good sprinkled onto meat before grilling, roasting or broiling.

- Cajun seasoning is a blend of red pepper, garlic, onion, salt, and pepper used to add a hot taste to any dish.

- Italian seasoning is a favorite mix of basil and oregano useful in most pasta dishes.

- Lemon pepper seasoning adds flavor to poultry and vegetables.

- Mexican seasoning contains a mixture of peppers, garlic, salt, and cumin suitable for tacos, fajitas, and enchiladas.

A great way to stock your pantry with spices is to buy one or two new ones each time you go shopping and buy fresh herbs only when needed.

Sauces

Sauces are a great way to add flavor to your dishes. Here are some sauces you should have on hand in your kitchen:

- Barbecue sauce

- Chili sauce

- Hot pepper sauce

- Olive oil

- Packages of dried onion soup mix

- Packages of salad dressing mix

- Soy sauce

- Soups in a can (cream of mushroom, chicken, celery)

- Steak sauce

- Sweet and sour sauce

- Teriyaki sauce

- Vinegar (red, rice, and balsamic)

- Wine (red and white suitable, for drinking)

- Worcestershire sauce

Basic Grocery Items

You also need some essential grocery items, things you will find yourself using over and over in myriad recipes. These kitchen basics include:

- Beans (a variety of canned and dried)

- Bread crumbs

- Bullion cubes and powders

- Cooking oil

- Crackers (a variety)

- Croutons

- Meats (canned tuna, chicken, crab, and clams)

- Olives (black and green)

- Pastas (a mixed variety)

- Rice (white, long grain, wild, brown)

- Salsa

- Tomatoes (a variety of canned)

- Tomato paste

- Tomato sauce

Baking Items

To bake like the best restaurants, you need to keep some baking basics in your pantry, including:

- Baking mix

- Baking powder

- Baking soda

- Brown sugar

- Confectioners' sugar

- Cocoa powder

- Cornstarch

- Flavored chips (chocolate, peanut butter, caramel)

- Flour

- Honey

- Nuts (a variety)

- Pancake mix

- Sugar

- Sweetened condensed milk

- Vegetable shortening

- Yeast

For Desserts

To create many restaurant-inspired desserts, you should have the following on hand:

- Applesauce

- Canned fruits

- Cake mixes, brownies, and frostings

- Fixings for ice cream sundaes

- Puddings

In the Refrigerator

Keep these items handy in the fridge so you can whip up your favorite copycat recipes without having to run out to the store. Make sure to have:

- Butter or margarine

- Cheeses (a good variety)

- Cream

- Eggs

- Ketchup

- Milk

- Mayonnaise

- Mustard

- Salad dressings

- Salad fixings (a variety of fresh vegetables)

- Sour cream

In the Freezer

There are a few items that, while you won't use them every day, you'll still want to keep stocked in your freezer. They include:

- Baguettes

- Boneless, skinless chicken breasts

- Bread and pizza dough

- Ground beef

- Steaks

- Stew meat

- Vegetables (broccoli, spinach, sliced green peppers)

With all these things on hand, you can put together a tasty and beautifully presented restaurant copycat meal in just a few minutes. The only thing you'll have to worry about is which recipe you want to try next.

Choosing Ingredients

Cooking from scratch always tastes better. Restaurant chefs seek out the freshest ingredients they can find and so should you. Skip the prepackaged items whenever you can. Generic brands may offer a lower price, but be careful to check out the quality and flavor — you may not be satisfied with the final taste of the dish. By upgrading your choices, you can turn an ordinary meal into something special. For example, instead of using plain iceberg lettuce try romaine or a spring mix, and don't settle for boring American cheese. Experiment and try new flavors.

Meats

Red meats should have a rosy bloom and poultry should look plump and moist. Meat packages should be firmly wrapped, with no leaking or excess moisture. Check expiration dates and package labeling to make sure that the meat is fresh and has been handled properly. Refrigerate meats as soon as they are purchased. Price is not always a reflection of quality; don't assume that the most expensive meat is the best.

Chicken

You can buy a whole chicken or in any variety of precut packages. The key to cooking with chicken is to be careful to avoid cross contamination and the risk of salmonella. Wash your hands and the chicken before cooking. Keep the uncooked chicken away from everything else on the kitchen counter. Use a separate cutting board and knife just for the uncooked chicken and do not use those same utensils for anything else. Clean anything the chicken touches thoroughly. If you follow these precautions, cooking with chicken is perfectly safe.

Beef

According to the USDA, ground beef cannot contain more than 30 percent fat by weight, so all of the packages will state their fat content. Get to know your butcher, and when London Broil or other roasts go on sale, have him grind it up for you to get premium ground beef at a reduced price.

How do you tell a great steak from a regular steak? The things to look for when buying a steak are the grade and the cut. Grade refers to the age of the animal and the marbling of the meat. The USDA grades the best steaks as prime, followed by choice and select. When selecting a steak, always take a look at the marbling or streaks of fat running through the meat. You want thin streaks that produce the best flavor. Cuts of steak are taken from different sections of the animal: The rib produces rib roast, back ribs, and rib eye steaks; the short loin produces the tastiest steaks like the T-bone, Porter-house, New York Strip, and the best cut of tenderloin.

ESSENTIAL

Always thaw meat in the refrigerator for maximum safety. Also, look for the safe handling label on packages of raw meat. It will tell you how to safely store, handle, and prepare meat and poultry.

Pork

All pork found in retail stores is inspected by the USDA. When buying pork, look for cuts with a relatively small amount of fat over the outside and with meat that is firm and grayish pink in color. For the best flavor, the meat should have a small amount of marbling. There are four basic cuts into which all other cuts are separated: the leg, side, loin, and shoulder. From those cuts, you get the bacon, ground pork for sausage, ribs, roasts, chops, and ham.

Fish

Knowing how to choose fresh fish is a skill all cooks should have. A fresh fish should smell like clean water. The eyes of the fish should be bright and clear and the gills should be a rich bright red. If it smells bad or looks discolored, don't buy it.

Fruits

Look for tenderness, plumpness, and bright color when choosing your fruit. Fruits should be heavy for their size and free of bruises, cuts, mildew, mold, or any other blemishes.

- Bananas are sold in any stage of ripeness and should be stored at room temperature.

- Berries should separate easily from their stems. Keep them refrigerated.

- Melons that have a sweet aromatic scent should be chosen. A strong smell indicates that they are overripe.

- Oranges, grapefruits, and lemons are sold when they are ripe. You may store them in the refrigerator for 2–3 weeks.

Vegetables

Take the time to inspect each vegetable before you buy. Look for crisp, plump, and brightly colored vegetables. Avoid the ones that are shriveled, bruised, moldy, or blemished.

- Asparagus should have straight stalks that are compact, with closed tips.

- Beans that are brightly colored and crisp are the best to select.

- Broccoli heads that are light green and yellowing should be avoided.

- Cabbage should have bright leaves without brown spots.

- Cauliflower with withered leaves and brown spots should not be chosen.

- Celery stalks should have firm crisp ribs.

- Cucumbers should be firm and not have soft spots.

- Peas that are shriveled or have brown spots should be avoided.

- Peppers that are crisp and bright colored should be chosen.

- Spinach leaves should be crisp and free of moisture.

Food Presentation

Whenever you go to an awesome restaurant, the vibes around that place become as important as the quality of the food served in determining whether or not you have a fulfilling experience. Remember that food presentation and table setting is of utmost value when serving a restaurant copycat meal.

Garnishes

The ingredients in the dish can pull double duty as garnishes. Save some fresh chopped herbs required in the dish to add just before plating. Use diced tomatoes or green onions on top of a dish. Shredded or shaved cheeses add a nice touch to almost any dish.

Plating

There are several types of plating techniques restaurants use, including:

- Pie style is where the plate is divided with a section for the protein, starch, and vegetables.

- The half-and-half style of plating is where the main dish is on one side of the plate with the accompaniments located on the other.

- Vertical plating is where you build the plate upward, usually with the protein on the bottom and the side dishes on top.

- Family style plating is where the food is served on large platters meant to be shared.

ESSENTIAL

Soup is such an inexpensive food to make at home. Why not splurge on some fancy oven-proof soup bowls to give a meal that special restaurant feeling with melted cheese on top?

Presenting Desserts

To showcase your beautifully created restaurant desserts, serve them in individual glass drinking glasses. A small wine glass layered with cake and ice cream or fruit and yogurt makes a nice presentation. Dessert shots are all the rage in the restaurants right now. Small sweet treats is a trend that's found its way onto dessert carts all over America. Little mini parfaits, sundaes, and layered cakes in shot glasses can easily be adapted for the home cook. It is time to raid your bar and fill those shot glasses with dessert. Small juice glasses also work well serving small-sized after-dinner treats.

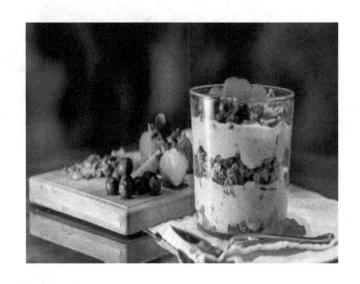

Breakfast

IHOP's Buttermilk Pancake

Preparation time: 5 minutes

Cooking time: 8 minutes

Servings: 8 to 10

Ingredients:

1¼ cups all-purpose flour

1 teaspoon baking soda

1 teaspoon baking powder

1¼ cups granulated sugar

1 pinch salt

1 egg

1¼ cups buttermilk

¼ cup cooking oil

Directions:

Preheat your pan by leaving it over medium heat while you are preparing the pancake batter.

Take all of your dry ingredients and mix them together.

Take all of your wet ingredients and mix them together.

Carefully combine the dry mixture into the wet mixture until everything is mixed together completely.

Melt some butter in your pan.

Slowly pour batter into the pan until you have a 5-inch circle.

Flip the pancake when its edges seem to have hardened.

Cook the other side of the pancake until it is golden brown.

Repeat steps six through eight until your batter is finished.

Serve with softened butter and maple syrup.

Nutrition: Calories 180.1, Total Fat 7.9 g, Carbs 23.2 g, Protein 4.1 g, Sodium 271.6 mg

McDonald's Breakfast Burrito

Preparation time: 10 minutes

Cooking time: 16 minutes

Servings: 10

Ingredients:

½ pound bulk sausage, cooked, crumbled

10 eggs, scrambled

1 medium tomato, diced

1 small onion, diced

3 tablespoons canned green chili, diced

Some salt and pepper

10 flour tortillas, warm

10 slices American cheese, halved

Some salsa

Some sour cream

Directions:

Mix the first six ingredients together in a medium-sized bowl.

Butter a non-stick pan over medium heat.

Pour the mixture into the pan and then cook until the egg is cooked the way you like.

When the mixture has reached your desired consistency, take it off the heat.

Lay out the tortillas and start assembling your burritos by placing one-tenth of the mixture in each of the tortillas.

Place the cheese on top of the egg mixture, then roll up the tortilla to make the burrito.

Garnish the roll with salsa and sour cream and serve.

Nutrition: Calories 270.1, Total Fat 14.8 g, Carbs 18.2 g, Protein 15.2 g, Sodium 525.3 mg

Starbucks's Marble Pound Cake

Preparation Time: 10 minutes

Cooking Time: 1 hour 30 minutes

Servings: 16

Ingredients:

4½ cups cake flour

2 teaspoons baking powder

⅛ teaspoon salt

6 ounces semisweet chocolate, finely chopped

2 cups unsalted butter, softened

3 cups granulated sugar

1 tablespoon vanilla

1 lemon, grated for zest

10 large eggs

2 tablespoons orange liquor OR milk

Directions:

Assemble your ingredients, and then:

a)   Preheat the oven to 350°F;

b)   Grease a 10×4-inch tube pan;

c)   Line the pan's bottom with greased wax paper; and

d)   Flour the entire pan.

Sift together the cake flour, baking powder, and salt in a medium-sized bowl—this is your dry mixture.

Melt the chocolate in a medium-sized bowl, then beat in the butter. When the mixture is smooth, beat in the sugar, lemon zest, and vanilla until the liquid mixture is uniform.

When the mixture is fully beaten, beat in the eggs, two at a time, until the mixture looks curdled.

Pour half of your dry mixture into your liquid mixture and mix until blended.

Add the orange liquor and the rest of the dry mixture. Continue beating the mixture.

When the mixture is blended, use a spatula to start folding it—this is your batter.

Set aside 4 cups of the batter. Whisk the melted chocolate into the remaining batter.

Now that you have a light batter and a dark batter, place the batter into the tube pan by the spoonful, alternating between the two colors.

When the pan is full, shake it slightly to level the batter. Run a knife through the batter to marble it.

Place the pan in the oven and bake for an hour and 15 minutes. To test if the cake is done, poke it with a toothpick. If there are still some moist crumbs on the toothpick when you take it out, then the cake is done.

Remove the cake from the pan and leave it to rest overnight.

Nutrition: Calories 582.1, Total Fat 32 g, Carbs 69.6 g, Protein 8.6 g, Sodium 114.8 mg

IHOP's Scrambled Egg

Preparation Time: 5 minutes

Cooking Time: 5 minutes

Servings: 4

Ingredients:

¼ cup pancake mix

1–2 tablespoons butter 6 large eggs

Salt and pepper, to taste

Directions:

Thoroughly beat the pancake mix and the eggs together until no lumps or clumps remain.

Butter a pan over medium heat.

When the pan is hot enough, pour the egg mixture in the middle of the pan.

Add the salt and pepper and let the mixture sit for about a minute.

When the egg starts cooking, start pushing the edges of the mixture toward the middle of the pan. Continue until the entire mixture is cooked.

Serve and enjoy.

Nutrition: Calories 870, Total Fat 54 g, Carbs 9 g, Protein 69 g, Sodium 34.9 mg

McDonald's' Fruit and Yogurt Parfait

Preparation Time: 5 minutes

Cooking Time: n/a

Servings: 10

Ingredients:

6 ounces vanilla yogurt, divided into 3

4–6 strawberries, sliced

¼ cup blueberries, fresh or frozen; divided into 2

¼ cup pecans, chopped; divided into 2

Directions:

Place 2 ounces of vanilla yogurt at the bottom of a cup, followed by 2–3 strawberries and ⅛ cup each of blueberries and pecans.

Place another layer of yogurt, strawberries, blueberries, and pecans on top of the first layer.

Finish off the parfait with the remaining yogurt—you can garnish it with more fruits if you like.

Nutrition: Calories 328.9, Total Fat 25.4 g, Carbs 20.7 g, Protein 9 g, Sodium 79.7 mg

Panera Bread's Cinnamon Crunch Bagel

Preparation Time: 1 hour

Cooking Time: 25 minutes

Servings: 8

Ingredients:

Bread:

1¼ cups warm water, between 110 to 120°F

1 tablespoon yeast

1 tablespoon salt

4 tablespoons honey, divided

1½ cups whole wheat pastry flour

½ tablespoon cinnamon

1¾ cups bread flour

¾ cup white chocolate chips

Cornmeal, for sprinkling

4¼ quarts water

Topping:

¼ cup granulated sugar

¼ cup packed brown sugar

1 tablespoon cinnamon

⅓ cup coconut oil

Directions:

Activate the yeast by mixing it with the warm water and setting it aside for 10 minutes.

Add in 3 tablespoons of the honey, the salt, the pastry flour, and the cinnamon. Mix all the ingredients together with a dough mixer or wooden spoon. After a minute of mixing, or when the flour is fully incorporated, scrape the sides of the bowl and mix again for another few minutes.

Let the dough rest for 5 minutes—if lumps form, stir the batter to break them apart.

Add in half a cup of bread flour and start kneading. Keep adding the bread flour half a cup at a time until it is finished, while kneading the dough to distribute the flour throughout.

After about seven minutes of kneading, add in the white chocolate chips and continue kneading to completely incorporate the chips into the mixture.

Cover the bowl with a towel and leave the dough to rest for one hour.

After an hour, flour a flat surface where you can place your dough. Transfer the dough from its bowl to the floured surface and punch it down.

Cut the dough into 8 equal pieces. Roll them into ropes. Let the dough rest again, for 3 to 4 minutes.

Form a circle with each piece of dough, twisting the ends securely together. Sprinkle a baking sheet with cornmeal and place the dough circles on the sheet. Cover with a towel and let rest for 10 to 15 minutes.

While the dough is resting, prepare your materials by:

(1) Bringing the water to a boil. When the water is boiling, add the remaining 1 tablespoon of honey. Keep the water at a low boil;

(2) Preheat the oven to 450°F;

(3) Line a baking sheet with parchment or wax paper; and

(4) Mix the topping ingredients (except the oil) together.

After 15 minutes, place a few dough circles into the boiling water. Leave them to cook for 50 seconds on each side. When the bagels have boiled, transfer them to the baking sheet using a slotted spoon so as to drain off the water.

When all the bagels have boiled, brush each one with coconut oil and sprinkle with the sugar mixture.

Bake your bagels for 20 to 25 minutes, then transfer them to a wire rack to let them cool.

Nutrition: Calories 463, Total Fat 16 g, Carbs 71 g, Protein 6 g, Sodium 296 mg

Starbucks's Chocolate Cinnamon Bread

Preparation Time: 15 minutes

Cooking Time: 1 hour

Servings: 16

Ingredients:

Bread:

1½ cups unsalted butter

3 cups granulated sugar

5 large eggs

2 cups flour

1¼ cups processed cocoa

1 tablespoon ground cinnamon

1 teaspoon salt

½ teaspoon baking powder

½ teaspoon baking soda

¼ cup water

1 cup buttermilk

1 teaspoon vanilla extract

Topping:

¼ cup granulated sugar

½ teaspoon cinnamon

½ teaspoon processed cocoa

⅛ teaspoon ginger, ground

⅛ teaspoon cloves, ground

Directions:

Before cooking:

a)   Preheat the oven to 350°F;

b)   Grease two 9×5×3 loaf pans; and

c)   Line the bottoms of the pans with wax paper.

Cream the sugar by beating it with the butter.

Beat the eggs into the mixture one at a time.

Sift the flour, cocoa, cinnamon, salt, baking powder, and baking soda into a large bowl.

In another bowl, whisk together the water, buttermilk, and vanilla.

Make a well in the dry mixture and start pouring in the wet mixtures a little at a time, while whisking.

When the mixture starts becoming doughy, divide it in two and transfer it to the pans.

Mix together all the topping ingredients and sprinkle evenly on top of the mixture in both pans.

Bake for 50 to 60 minutes, or until the bread has set.

Nutrition: Calories 370, Total Fat 14 g, Carbs 59 g, Protein 7 g, Sodium 270 mg

Starbucks's Lemon Loaf

Preparation Time: 15 minutes

Cooking Time: 45 minutes

Servings: 8

Ingredients:

Bread:

1½ cups flour

½ teaspoon baking soda

½ teaspoon baking powder

½ teaspoon salt

1 cup sugar

3 eggs, room temperature

2 tablespoons butter, softened

1 teaspoon vanilla extract

⅓ cup lemon juice

½ cup oil

Icing:

1 cup + 1 tablespoon powdered sugar

2 tablespoons milk

½ teaspoon lemon extract

Directions:

Get your baking materials ready by:

a) Preheating your oven to 350°F;

b) Greasing and flouring a 9×5×3 loaf pan; and

c) Lining pan's bottom with wax paper.

Mix the first four ingredients in a large bowl—this is your dry mixture.

Beat the eggs, butter, vanilla, and lemon juice together in a medium bowl until the mixture becomes smooth. This is your wet mixture.

Make a well in the middle of the dry mixture and pour the wet mixture into the well.

Mix everything together with a whisk or your hand mixer. Add the oil. Do not stop mixing until everything is fully blended and smooth.

Pour the batter into the pan and bake it for 45 minutes—the bread is ready when you can stick a toothpick into it and it comes out clean.

While the bread is baking, make the icing by mixing the icing ingredients in a small bowl using a whisk or hand mixer until smooth.

When the bread is done baking, place it on a cooling rack and leave it for at least 20 minutes to cool.

When the bread is cool enough, pour the icing over the top. Wait for the icing to set before slicing.

Nutrition: Calories 425.2, Total Fat 18.7 g, Carbs 60 g, Protein 5 g, Sodium 310.8 mg

Waffle House's Waffle

Preparation Time: 5 minutes

Cooking Time: 20 minutes

Servings: 6

Ingredients:

1½ cups all-purpose flour

1 teaspoon salt

½ teaspoon baking soda

1 egg

½ cup + 1 tablespoon granulated white sugar

2 tablespoons butter, softened

2 tablespoons shortening

½ cup half-and-half

½ cup milk

¼ cup buttermilk

¼ teaspoon vanilla

Directions:

Prepare the dry mixture by sifting the flour into a bowl and mixing it with the salt and baking soda.

In a medium bowl, lightly beat an egg. When the egg has become frothy, beat in the butter, sugar, and shortening. When the mixture is thoroughly mixed, beat in the half-and-half, vanilla, milk, and buttermilk. Continue beating the mixture until it is smooth.

While beating the wet mixture, slowly pour in the dry mixture, making sure to mix thoroughly and remove all the lumps.

Chill the batter overnight (optional, but recommended; if you can't chill the mixture overnight, leave it for at least 15 to 20 minutes).

Take the batter out of the refrigerator. Preheat and grease your waffle iron.

Cook each waffle for three to four minutes. Serve with butter and syrup.

Nutrition: Calories 313.8, Total Fat 12.4 g, Carbs 45 g, Protein 5.9 g, Sodium 567.9 mg

Mimi's Café Santa Fé Omelet

Preparation Time: 10 minutes

Cooking Time: 10 minutes

Servings: 1

Ingredients:

Chipotle Sauce:

1 cup marinara or tomato sauce

¾ cup water

½ cup chipotle in adobo sauce

1 teaspoon kosher salt

Omelet:

1 tablespoon onions, diced

1 tablespoon jalapeños, diced

2 tablespoons cilantro, chopped

2 tablespoons tomatoes, diced

¼ cup fried corn tortillas, cut into strips

3 eggs, beaten

2 slices cheese

1 dash of salt and pepper

Garnish:

2 ounces chipotle sauce, hot

¼ cup fried corn tortillas, cut into strips

1 tablespoon sliced green onions

1 tablespoon guacamole

Directions:

Melt some butter in a pan over medium heat, making sure to coat the entire pan.

Sauté the jalapeños, cilantro, tomatoes, onions, and tortilla strips for about a minute.

Add the eggs, seasoning them with salt and pepper and stirring occasionally.

Flip the omelet when it has set. Place the cheese on the top half.

When the cheese starts to become melty, fold the omelet in half and transfer to a plate.

Garnish the omelet with chipotle sauce, guacamole, green onions, and corn tortillas.

Nutrition: Calories 519, Total Fat 32 g, Carbs 60 g, Protein 14 g, Sodium 463 mg

Appetizers

Southwestern Egg Rolls

Preparation Time: 10 minutes

Cooking Time: 10 minutes

Servings: 6

Ingredients:

For Smoked Chicken Ingredients:

8 ounces chicken breast

1 teaspoon vegetable oil or olive oil

Egg Roll filling:

½ cup canned black beans, rinsed & drained

¼ cup red bell peppers, minced

2 teaspoons pickled jalapeno peppers, chopped

½ cup frozen corn

8 flour tortillas (7" each)

¼ cup spinach, frozen, thawed & drained

1 teaspoon taco seasoning

¾ cup Monterey jack cheese, shredded

1 tablespoon vegetable oil or olive oil

¼ cup green onions, minced

Avocado Ranch Ingredients

½ cup milk

1 package Ranch dressing mix

½ cup mayonnaise

¼ cup fresh avocados, smashed (approximately half of an avocado)

For Toppings:

1 tablespoon onions, chopped

2 tablespoons tomatoes, chopped

Directions:

For Chicken Breast:

Preheat grill over moderate heat. Generously season the chicken pieces with black pepper and salt. Brush the chicken breast with vegetable or olive oil. Grill over the preheated hot grill; cook for 5 to 7 minutes per side. Chop the chicken into small pieces; set aside until ready to use.

For Egg roll filling:

Sauté the red pepper for a couple of minutes, until just become tender. Add the corn, green onion, pickled jalapenos, and black beans to the mixture. Add in the taco seasoning; continue to cook until heated through.

Place equal amounts of filing, equal portions of chicken into the tortillas & top with the cheese. Fold in the ends & tightly roll them up. Secure your wrapped tortillas with toothpicks.

For Egg Rolls

Fill a large pot with vegetable oil (enough to cover the bottom by 4") and then heat it over moderate heat. Once hot; deep fry the egg rolls for 7 to 8 minutes in total, until turn golden brown. When done; immediately remove them from the hot oil & arrange them on a wire rack.

For Avocado Ranch Dressing

Prepare the Ranch dressing mix with ½ cup of buttermilk & ½ cup mayonnaise. Add approximately ¼ cup of the mashed avocado into the mixture. Add the mixture in a blender and pulse on high for a minute, until blended well.

Nutrition: Calories: 123, Fat: 23 g, Carbs: 46 g, Protein: 16 g, Sodium: 87

Skillet Queso

Preparation Time: 5 minutes

Cooking Time: 15 minutes

Servings: 4

Ingredients:

16 ounce box Velveeta cheese; cut into cubes

½ teaspoon ground cayenne pepper

2 teaspoons paprika

1 cups milk

15 ounce can Hormel Chili No Beans

Juice of 1 medium lime, freshly squeezed (approximately 1 tablespoon)

4 teaspoons chili powder

½ teaspoon ground cumin

Directions:

Over medium heat in a medium saucepan; combine the cheese together with the leftover ingredients. Cook for a couple of minutes, until the cheese melts completely, stirring frequently to prevent sticking.

Serve the queso with tortilla chips and enjoy.

Nutrition: Calories:533, Fat:25 g, Carbs: 47 g, Protein: 12 g, Sodium:1129 mg

White Spinach Queso

Preparation Time: 5 minutes

Cooking Time: 10 minutes

Servings: 12

Ingredients:

2 tablespoons flour

8 ounces white American cheese

2 cups baby spinach leaves, fresh

¾ cup whole milk

2 tablespoons butter

½ teaspoon garlic powder

2 cups Jack cheese

1 tablespoon canola oil

Optional Ingredients:

Queso fresco crumbles

Pico de Gallo salsa

Guacamole

Directions:

Set your oven to broil. Now, over medium high heat in a large, cast iron skillet; heat the canola oil until hot. Add and cook the spinach until just wilted; immediately remove from the hot pan.

Add butter to the hot pan and then add the flour, stir well & cook for a few seconds then slowly add the milk.

Add in the garlic powder; whisk well then add the cheeses.

Continue to stir the mixture until thick & bubbly, for a minute or two and then, add in the spinach leaves; stir well.

Broil until the top turn golden brown, for a couple of minutes.

Top with salsa, guacamole and queso; serve immediately & enjoy.

Nutrition: Calories: 459, Fat: 15 g, Carbs: 67 g, Protein: 15 g, Sodium: 1008 mg

Awesome Blossom Petals

Preparation Time:15 minutes

Cooking Time: 15 minutes

Servings: 6

Ingredients:

For Seasoned Breading:

¼ teaspoon onion powder

2 ½ cups flour

½ teaspoon ground black pepper

2 teaspoons seasoned salt

½ teaspoon paprika

1 cup buttermilk

¼ teaspoon garlic powder

For Blossom Sauce:

1/8 teaspoon cayenne pepper

2 tablespoons ketchup

½ cup sour cream

1 ½ teaspoons prepared horseradish

½ teaspoon seasoned salt

Other ingredients:

vegetable oil for frying

Directions:

For Blossom Sauce:

Combine the sour cream with ketchup, horseradish, cayenne pepper and seasoned salt in a small bowl; stir the ingredients well. Cover & let chill in a refrigerator until ready to serve.

For Onion:

Peel the onion.

Cut the stem of the onion off; place it on the cutting board, stem side down. Cut the onion horizontally and vertically into half then make two more diagonal cuts.

For Breading:

Add buttermilk in a large bowl.

Combine flour together with garlic powder, black pepper, paprika, onion powder and seasoned salt in a separate bowl. Using a large fork; give the ingredients a good stir until well mixed.

Put the onions first into the flour and then dip them into the buttermilk; then into the flour again. Let the onions to rest on the wire rack.

For Cooking:

Preheat oil until it reaches 350 F. Work in batches & add the onions into the hot oil (ensure that you don't overcrowd the onions); cook until turn golden brown, for 2 to 3 minutes.

Remove them from the hot oil & then place them on a wire rack to drain.

Serve hot & enjoy.

Nutrition: Calories: 158, Fat: 5 g, Carbs: 20 g, Protein:17 g

Chili's Buffalo wings

Preparation Time: 5 minutes

Cooking Time: 25 minutes

Servings: 2

Ingredients:

1 cup all-purpose flour

¼ cup hot sauce

1 cup 1% milk

¼ teaspoon paprika

5 cup vegetable oil

1 organic egg, large

2 chicken breast fillets; sliced into six pieces

1 tablespoon margarine

½ teaspoon black pepper

2 teaspoon salt

¼ teaspoon cayenne pepper

Directions:

In a large-sized mixing bowl; combine flour together with paprika, peppers and salt; mix well & set aside. Whisk the egg together with milk in a separate small-sized mixing bowl. Now, over moderate heat in a large, deep fryer; heat up 5 cups of the vegetable oil.

Dip each of your chicken pieces into the egg mixture and then into the breading blend. Continue to dip the pieces for one more time and ensure that all pieces are coated well. Set them on a plate to chill for 10 to 15 minutes.

Once done; carefully add the chicken pieces into the hot oil & fry until turn crispy & golden brown, for 4 to 5 minutes. In the meantime; combine the margarine with hot sauce in a separate mixing bowl & microwave until the margarine is melted, for 25 seconds.

When you are done with the chicken pieces; place them on a paper towel lined plate. Once done; place the chicken pieces into a plastic container & add the prepared sauce.

Close the container; shake well until the chicken is completely covered with the sauce. Serve immediately & enjoy.

Nutrition: Calories: 323, Fat: 34 g, Carbs: 7g, Protein:35 g, Sodium: 357 mg

Loaded Boneless Wings

Preparation Time: 30 minutes

Cooking Time: 50 minutes

Servings: 10

Ingredients:

For Veggie Queso Dip:

1 jalapeno pepper, finely chopped

½ yellow bell pepper, finely chopped

¼ teaspoon ground cumin

1 package American cheese, shredded (6 ounce)

½ red bell pepper, finely chopped

2 slices of Fontana cheese, shredded

½ teaspoon red pepper flakes

1 ball mozzarella cheese, shredded (4 ounce)

½ teaspoon olive oil

1/8 teaspoon each of garlic powder, ground black pepper, onion powder, ground nutmeg & salt

½ cup half-and-half

For Wings:

4 strips of bacon or to taste

1 package Buffalo-style boneless chicken breast halves, frozen (25.5 ounce)

½ pound cheddar cheese, shredded

3 green onions, thinly sliced

¼ pound Monterey Jack cheese, shredded

Directions:

Over medium heat in a large skillet; heat the olive oil until hot. Once done; add the yellow bell pepper together with red bell pepper & jalapeno pepper; stir well & cook for 2 to 3 minutes, until mostly tender, stirring constantly. Add the cumin; cook & stir for a minute more, until the peppers are nicely coated. Add half-&-half; let simmer until almost boiling. Decrease the heat to low and slowly stir in the mozzarella cheese, fontina cheese, American cheese, red pepper flakes, onion powder, garlic powder, nutmeg, black pepper and salt. Cook for 3 to 5 more minutes, until the cheeses are melted completely, stirring constantly.

Preheat oven to 400 F.

Place the frozen chicken breasts on a large-sized baking sheet & the bacon strips on a separate sheet.

Place both the pans in the preheated oven. Heat the chicken for 10 to 12 minutes, until thawed; remove from the oven. Continue to bake the bacon for 16 to 18 more minutes, until crispy. Leave the oven on; remove the bacon, place it on a paper towel to dry & then chop into pieces.

Place a cup of the prepared queso dip into the bottom of a large ovenproof dish or skillet. Arrange the chicken over the top & sprinkle with Monterey Jack cheese and Cheddar cheese.

Bake for 5 to 8 more minutes, until the cheeses have completely melted. Sprinkle with the chopped green onion and bacon pieces.

Nutrition: Calories: 377, Fat: 34 g, Carbs: 62 g, Protein: 21 g, Sodium: 647 mg

Classic Nachos

Preparation Time: 25 minutes

Cooking Time: 2 hours and 15 minutes

Servings: 5 persons

Ingredients:

2 tablespoon guacamole

1 boneless chicken breast, uncooked, cut in strips

A bag of tortilla chips, any of your choice

1 cup fresh lettuce, shredded

½ cup Monterey Jack cheese, shredded

1 package of fajita seasoning mix (1 ounces)

½ cup sharp cheddar cheese, shredded

1 jalapeño, sliced

½ cup your choice salsa

1 Vidalia onion, sliced

2 tablespoon low-fat sour cream

1 bell pepper, sliced

Directions:

Over moderate heat in a large skillet; sauté the chicken with onion, fajita seasoning & peppers. When done; drain the prepared fajita mixture & set aside until ready to use.

Now, spread the tortillas out on your ovenproof platter in a large circle. Once done; start layering them with chicken, peppers and onions. Add the cheeses followed by the jalapenos. Place the platter into the oven & bake until the cheese is completely melted, for 5 to 10 minutes, at 350 F. Once done; pull out the platter & add the shredded lettuce in the center of chip circle. Top the lettuce with sour cream, salsa & guacamole. Serve immediately & enjoy.

Nutrition: Calories: 345, Fat: 14 g, Carbs: 34 g, Protein:54 g, Sodium: 1435 mg

Fried Pickles

Preparation Time: 5 minutes

Cooking Time: 10 minutes

Servings: 4

Ingredients:

2 cup pickle chips

¼ teaspoon cayenne pepper

1 teaspoon sugar

½ teaspoon pepper

2 cup flour

Oil, for frying

1 teaspoon salt

Directions:

Over moderate heat in a deep pan; heat the oil until hot. Now, in a large bowl; combine the flour together with cayenne, sugar, pepper, and salt; continue to whisk until combined well.

Drain the pickle chips & then toss them into the prepared flour mixture. Once done, work in batches and fry them (ensure that you don't overcrowd the pan). Once the pickles starts to float to the surface, immediately remove them from the hot oil. Place them on paper towels to drain; serve with the horseradish or ranch dressing and enjoy.

Nutrition: Calories: 266, Fat: 20 g, Carbs: 34 g, Protein: 23 g, Sodium: 624 mg

Crispy Cheddar Bites

Preparation Time: 15 minutes

Cooking Time: 20 minutes

Servings: 4

Ingredients:

1 cup all-purpose flour

½ cup softened butter, at room temperature (1 stick)

1 cup sharp cheddar cheese, shredded, slightly packed

1/8 teaspoon cayenne pepper

1 cup crispy rice cereal

¼ teaspoon salt

Directions:

Preheat oven to 375 F. Lightly coat two rimmed baking sheets with the cooking spray.

Using a wooden spoon; combine the entire ingredients together in a large bowl; continue to mix until thoroughly mixed. Make 1" balls from the prepared mixture & arrange them on coated baking sheets. Slightly flatten the balls using the bottom of a drinking glass or the palm of your hand.

Bake in the preheated oven until the edges turn golden brown, for 10 to 12 minutes. Serve warm & enjoy.

Nutrition: Calories: 366, Fat: 25 g, Carbs: 45 g, Protein:42 g, Sodium: 428 mg

Texas Chili Fries

Preparation Time: 10 minutes

Cooking Time: 20 minutes

Servings: 4

Ingredients:

1 package of bacon

1 bag cheese blend, shredded

Ranch salad dressing

1 bag steak fries, frozen

1 jar jalapeno peppers

Directions:

Evenly spread the fries over a large-sized cookie sheet & bake as per the directions mentioned on the package.

Line strips of bacon on a separate cookie sheet & bake until crispy.

When the bacon and fries are done; remove them from the oven.

Add a thick layer of jalapenos and cheese; crumble the bacon over the fries.

Bake in the oven again until the cheese is completely melted.

Serve hot with some Ranch salad dressing on side and enjoy.

Nutrition: Calories: 537, Fat: 17 g, Carbs: 56 g, Protein: 36 g, Sodium: 683 mg

Chili's Salad

Preparation Time: 25 minutes

Cooking Time: 15 minutes

Servings: 4

Ingredients:

For Pico De Gallo:

2 teaspoon seeded jalapeno peppers, finely diced

½ cup red onion finely minced

2 medium tomatoes diced very small

2 teaspoon cilantro, fresh & finely minced

For Salad:

4 chicken breasts skinless, boneless

5 ounces bag half-and-half spring mix with baby spinach

½ cup red cabbage chopped

6.5 ounces bag butter bliss lettuce or romaine or iceberg lettuce

¾ cup craisins

1 cup fresh pineapple chunked

¼ cup teriyaki sauce

14 ounces can mandarin orange segments drained

Tortilla strips

¼ cup water

For Honey-Lime Dressing:

1 cup vanilla Greek yogurt

¼ cup Dijon mustard

1 tablespoon lime juice, freshly squeezed

3 tablespoon apple cider vinegar

1 cup honey

2 tablespoon sesame oil

½ to 1 teaspoon lime zest grated

Directions:

For Pico De Gallo:

Combine the ingredients for Pico de Gallo together in a small bowl & let chill in a refrigerator until ready to use.

For Salad:

1. Mix the teriyaki sauce with water.

Place the chicken pieces in a large-sized plastic bag or plastic bowl.

Add in the prepared teriyaki mixture & let marinate for an hour or two in the refrigerator.

Layer the lettuce & spring mix in large serving bowl.

Add craisins and cabbage; toss well.

Refrigerate until all ingredients are ready.

After chicken has marinated; lightly coat your grill with the cooking spray and heat it over moderate heat.

Remove the chicken pieces from marinade; shaking off any excess.

Add to the hot grill & cook until the chicken is cooked through, for 5 to 10 minutes on each side.

Slice chicken down into cubes or thin strips. Set aside on the serving plate to serve.

For Honey-Lime Dressing:

Combine the entire salad dressing ingredients in a blender; blend on high until blended well.

Refrigerate until ready to serve.

To Assemble the Salad:

Remove the salad to four individual large serving plates.

Place approximately ¼ cup of the mandarin orange segments & pineapple over each salad.

Sprinkle with the chicken.

Top with a spoonful or two of Pico de Gallo or to taste.

Drizzle with salad dressing; give the ingredients a good stir until mixed well.

Garnish with the tortilla strips. Serve immediately & enjoy.

Nutrition: Calories: 535, Fat: 33 g, Carbs: 24 g, Protein: 51 g, Sodium: 635 mg

Raspberry Lemonade

Preparation Time: 2 minutes

Cooking Time: 3 minutes

Servings: 8

Ingredients:

1 cup water

1 cup sugar

1 cup freshly squeezed lemon juice

1 ½ cups fresh or frozen raspberries

Extra sugar for the rim of your glass

Directions:

In a small saucepan, heat the water and sugar until the sugar completely dissolves.

Meanwhile, purée the raspberries in a blender. Add the contents of the saucepan and the cup of lemon juice. (If it's too thick you can add extra water.)

Wet the rim of your glass and dip it into a bit of sugar to coat the rim before pouring the lemonade into the glass.

Nutrition: Calories: 234, Fat: 56. 2 g, Carbs: 23. 8 g, Protein: 23. 5 g, Sodium: 1324 mg

Lunch (Chicken)

Alice Springs Chicken from Outback

Preparation Time: 5 minutes

Cooking Time: 2 hours and 30 minutes

Servings: 4

Ingredients:

Sauce:

½ cup Dijon mustard

½ cup honey

¼ cup mayonnaise

1 teaspoon fresh lemon juice

Chicken preparation:

4 chicken breast, boneless and skinless

2 tablespoons butter

1 tablespoon olive oil

8 ounces fresh mushrooms, sliced

4 slices bacon, cooked and cut into 2-inch pieces

2 ½ cups Monterrey Jack cheese, shredded

Parsley for serving (optional)

Directions:

Preheat oven to 400 °F.

Mix together ingredients for the sauce in a bowl.

Put chicken in a Ziploc bag, then add sauce into bag until only ¼ cup is left. Keep remaining sauce in a container, cover, and refrigerate. Make sure to seal Ziploc bag tightly and shake gently until chicken is coated with sauce Keep in refrigerator for at least 2 hours.

Melt butter in a pan over medium heat. Toss in mushrooms and cook for 5 minutes or until brown. Remove from pan and place on a plate.

In an oven-safe pan, heat oil. Place marinated chicken flat in pan and cook for 5 minutes on each side or until both sides turn golden brown.

Nutrition: Calories: 888, Fat: 56 g, Carbs: 41 g, Protein: 59 g, Sodium: 1043 mg

Panda Express' Orange Chicken

Preparation Time: 15 minutes

Cooking Time: 30 minutes

Servings: 6

Ingredients:

Orange sauce:

1½ tablespoon soy sauce

1½ tablespoon water

5 tablespoons sugar

5 tablespoons white vinegar

3 tablespoons orange zest

Chicken preparation:

1 egg - 1½ teaspoon salt

White pepper, to taste

5 tablespoons grapeseed oil, divided

½ cup + 1 tablespoon cornstarch

¼ cup flour

¼ cup cold water

2 pounds chicken breast, boneless and skinless, chopped

1 teaspoon fresh ginger, grated

1 teaspoon garlic, finely chopped

½ teaspoon hot red chili pepper, ground

¼ cup green onion, sliced - 1 tablespoon rice wine

½ teaspoon sesame oil

White rice and steamed broccoli for serving

Directions:

Mix together ingredients for the orange sauce in a bowl. Reserve for later.

Add egg, salt, pepper, and 1 tablespoon oil to a separate bowl. Mix well.

In another bowl, combine ½ cup cornstarch and flour. Mix until fully blended.

Add remaining cornstarch and cold water in a different bowl. Blend until cornstarch is completely dissolved.

Heat 3 tablespoons oil in a large deep skillet or wok over high heat.

Coat chicken pieces in egg mixture. Let excess drip off. Then, coat in cornstarch mixture. Cook for at least 3 minutes or until both sides are golden brown and chicken is cooked through. Arrange on a plate lined with paper towels to drain excess oil.

In a clean large deep skillet, or wok heat remaining oil on high heat. Lightly sauté ginger and garlic for 30 seconds or until aromatic. Toss in peppers and green onions. Stir-fry vegetables for 1-3 minutes, then pour in rice wine. Mix well before adding orange sauce. Bring to a boil. Mix in cooked chicken pieces, then add cornstarch mixture. Simmer until mixture is thick, then mix in sesame oil.

Transfer onto a plate and serve with white rice and steamed broccoli.

Nutrition: Calories: 305, Fat: 5 g, Carbs: 27 g, Protein: 34 g, Sodium: 1024 mg

Chili's Boneless Buffalo Wings

Preparation Time: 30 minutes

Cooking Time: 15 minutes

Servings: 2

Ingredients:

1 cup flour

2 teaspoons salt

½ teaspoon black pepper, ground

¼ teaspoon cayenne pepper, ground

1 egg

1 cup milk

5 cups vegetable oil

2 chicken breasts, boneless and skinless, cut into 6 pieces

¼ cup hot sauce

1 tablespoon margarine

1 blue cheese salad dressing

1 stalk celery, cut into sticks

Directions:

In a bowl, mix together flour, salt, peppers, and paprika.

Add egg and milk to a separate bowl and mix well.

Preheat 5 cups oil in a deep-fryer to 375 °F.

Coat chicken pieces into egg mixture. Allow excess to drip off, then coat with flour mixture. Repeat twice for a double coat.

Transfer breaded chicken onto a plate and refrigerate for about 15 minutes.

Deep-fry each for about 5 minutes or until brown and transfer onto a paper towel-lined plate.

Meanwhile, mix hot sauce and margarine in a bowl. Then, heat in the microwave for about 20 seconds or until melted. Mix well until fully blended.

Place chicken pieces in a large Ziploc bag and add sauce. Seal bag tightly. Using your hands, mix chicken and sauce together until well-coated.

Serve chicken pieces on a plate with blue cheese dressing and celery sticks on the side.

Nutrition: Calories: 398, Fat: 13 g, Carbs: 55 g, Protein: 14 g, Sodium: 3234 mg

Boston Market's Rotisserie Chicken Copycat

Preparation Time: 24 hours

Cooking Time: 1 hour

Servings: 4

Ingredients:

¼ cup apple cider vinegar

½ cup canola oil

2 tablespoons brown sugar

4 fresh garlic cloves, finely chopped

1 whole roasting chicken

Directions:

Combine vinegar, oil, sugar, and garlic in a bowl. Add chicken and spoon mixture on top to coat well. Refrigerate overnight, making sure to turn chicken over to soak opposite side

Remove chicken from refrigerator. Set aside for at least 20 minutes.

Bake at 350°F for about 45-50 minutes or until the temperature reads 165°F on an instant meat thermometer inserted in thickest part of the thigh without touching any bones.

Serve.

Nutrition: Calories: 433, Fat: 39 g, Carbs: 8 g, Protein: 13 g, Sodium: 53 mg

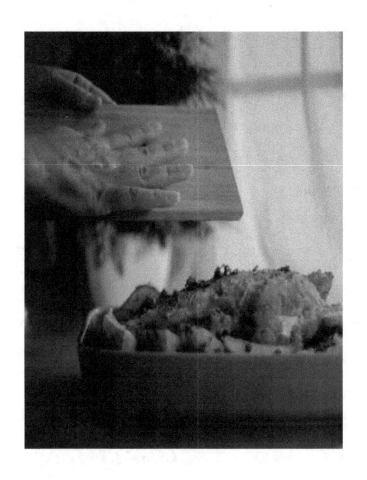

Cracker Barrel Chicken and Dumplings

Preparation Time: 1 hour

Cooking Time: 2 hours

Servings: 6

Ingredients:

1 whole chicken

2 quarts water

2 teaspoons salt

½ teaspoon pepper

2 cups all-purpose flour

½ teaspoon baking soda

½ teaspoon salt

3 tablespoons shortening

¾ cup buttermilk

Directions:

In a heavy bottomed pot, boil chicken in water mixed with salt. Cover, then lower heat. Simmer for about 1 hour or until tender enough that the meat almost falls off the bone.

Using a slotted spoon, transfer chicken to a plate and cool. Then, remove bones and chop into small pieces.

In same pot, add broth and bring to a boil Add pepper.

In a bowl, mix flour, baking soda, and salt. Fold in shortening. Pour in buttermilk and mix everything until incorporated.

Knead dough 4 to 5 times. Pinch off about ½ inch size balls of dough and to the boiling broth. Reduce heat to medium-low. Simmer for about 8 to 10 minutes while stirring every now and then.

Add chicken to pot and stir.

Serve immediately.

Nutrition: Calories: 711, Fat: 41 g, Saturated fat: 12 g, Carbs: 33 g, Sugar: 2 g, Fibers: 1 g, Protein: 48 g, Sodium: 1276 mg

Chipotle's Chicken

Preparation Time: 10 minutes

Cooking Time: 20 minutes

Marinate Time: 24 hours

Servings: 8

Ingredients:

2 ½ pound organic boneless and skinless chicken breasts or thighs

Olive oil or cooking spray

Marinade

7 oz. chipotle peppers in adobo sauce

2 tablespoons olive oil

6 garlic cloves, peeled

1 teaspoon black pepper

2 teaspoons salt

½ teaspoon cumin

½ teaspoon dry oregano

Directions:

Pour all the marinade ingredients in a food processor or blender and blend until you get a smooth paste.

Pound the chicken until it has a thickness between ½ to ¾ inch. Place chicken into an airtight container or re-sealable plastic bag such as a Ziploc. Pour the marinade over the chicken and stir until well coated. Place the chicken in the refrigerator and let marinate overnight or up to 24 hours.

Pour the blended mixture into the container and marinate the chicken for at least 8 hours.

Cook the chicken over medium to high heat on an oiled and preheated grill for 3 to 5 minutes per side. The internal temperature of the chicken should be 165°F before you remove it from the heat. You can also cook it in heavy bottomed skillet over medium heat with a little olive oil.

Let rest before serving. If desired, cut into cubes to add to salads, tacos or quesadillas or serve as is.

Nutrition: Calories: 293, Fat: 18.7 g, Carbs: 5.8 g, Protein: 24.9 g, Sodium: 526 mg

Popeye's Fried Chicken

Preparation Time: 20 minutes

Cooking Time: 45 minutes

Servings: 8

Ingredients:

Breading:

3 cups self-rising flour

1 cup corn starch

3 tablespoons seasoning salt

2 tablespoons paprika

1 teaspoon baking soda

1 package (0.7 ounce) dry Italian-style salad dressing mix

1 package (1 ounce) dry onion soup mix

1 (1 ½ ounces) packet dry spaghetti sauce spices and seasoning mix

3 tablespoons white sugar

Batter/Coating:

3 cups cornflakes cereal, crushed

2 eggs, beaten

¼ cup cold water

Chicken:

2 cups oil for frying

1 (4-pound) whole chicken, cut into pieces

Directions:

Mix all of the breading ingredients together in a deep bowl.

Place the crushed cereal in another bowl.

In another bowl, beat the eggs and cold water together.

Heat the oil to 350°F and preheat the oven to 350°F.

Dip the chicken into the breading mixture, the egg mixture, the crushed cereal, and then the breading mixture again.

Immediately place the breaded chicken into the heated oil and cook on each side for 3 to 4 minutes.

Place the chicken in a 9×13 baking pan skin-side up. Cover the baking pan with foil, leaving a small opening.

Bake the chicken for 45 minutes.

After 45 minutes, remove the foil and continue baking for another 5 minutes.

Remove the baking pan from the oven and serve.

Nutrition: Calories: 733, Fat: 26.8 g, Carbs: 76.3 g, Protein: 44.3 g, Sodium: 3140 mg

McDonald's Chicken Nuggets

Preparation Time: 45 minutes

Cooking Time: 45 minutes

Servings: 4

Ingredients:

Chicken:

1 pound chicken tenderloins, boneless and thawed

Brine:

4 cups water, cold

2 teaspoons fine sea salt

Breading:

⅓ + ½ cup all-purpose flour, sifted

All-purpose flour, sifted

½ cup corn starch

1½ tablespoons seasoned salt

1 tablespoon fine corn flour

1½ teaspoons dry milk powder, non-fat

1 teaspoon granulated sugar

½ teaspoon ginger, ground

¼ teaspoon mustard, ground

¼ teaspoon black pepper, fine

¼ teaspoon white pepper, fine

⅛ teaspoon allspice, ground

⅛ teaspoon cloves, ground

⅛ teaspoon paprika, ground

⅛ teaspoon turmeric, ground

1 pinch cinnamon, ground

1 pinch cayenne pepper

Batter:

2 eggs, beaten

½ cup water, cold

2 tablespoons corn starch

2 tablespoons all-purpose flour

¼ teaspoon sea salt, fine

¼ teaspoon sesame oil

¼ teaspoon soy sauce

¼ teaspoon granulated sugar

For Deep Frying:

Vegetable oil, 3 parts

Vegetable shortening, 1 part

Directions:

Pound the chicken until it is only ½ inch thick.

Mix the brine ingredients.

Cut the chicken into small, chicken-nugget-sized pieces and place them in the brine. Leave it in the refrigerator for 2 hours.

When the chicken is almost done soaking, whisk together all the batter ingredients. Also mix together all the breading ingredients.

Remove the chicken from the refrigerator and evenly coat each piece with the batter.

Evenly coat each battered piece with the breading.

Slowly heat the deep-frying ingredients to 350°F.

Deep fry each nugget and then transfer to a plate with a paper towel to drain the oil.

Transfer to a different plate and serve.

Note: The nuggets can be battered up and breaded in advance and stored in an airtight container if you want to fry them later

Nutrition: Calories: 370.5, Fat: 5 g, Carbs: 44.9 g, Protein: 33.2 g, Sodium: 1457.4 m

Ruby Tuesday's Sonora Chicken Pasta

Preparation Time: 25 minutes

Cooking Time: 20 minutes

Servings: 4

Ingredients:

Cheese Mixture

1 pound processed cheese like Velveeta

½ cup heavy cream

2 teaspoons olive oil

2 tablespoons red chili peppers, minced

2 tablespoons green chili peppers, minced

2 tablespoons onions, minced

½ garlic clove, minced

2 tablespoons water

¼ teaspoon salt

2 teaspoons sugar

½ tablespoon vinegar

¼ teaspoon cumin

Beans:

1 can 15-ounce can black beans, with the water

2 tablespoons green chili peppers, minced

2 tablespoons onions, minced

½ garlic clove, minced

¼ teaspoon salt

1 dash paprika

Seasoning and Chicken:

Vegetable oil

½ teaspoon salt

1 dash dried thyme

1 dash dried summer savory

4 chicken breast halves, boneless, skinless

Pasta:

1 box (16 ounces) penne pasta

4 quarts water

1 tablespoon butter

Garnish:

Green onion, chopped

Tomatoes, diced

Directions:

Preheat your grill.

Mix the Velveeta and the cream over heat until smooth.

In another pan, heat the olive oil and sauté the peppers, onions, and garlic clove.

After 2 minutes, add the water and bring to a simmer for another 2 minutes.

Add the sautéed vegetables to the cheese and continue simmering over low heat. Add in the salt, the sugar, the vinegar, and the cumin, and leave the entire mixture over low heat. Make sure to stir.

In another saucepan, bring the beans, peppers, onions, garlic, salt, and paprika to a boil over medium heat.

When the bean mixture starts boiling, reduce the heat to low and keep it simmering.

Mix all the seasoning ingredients and then rub the seasoning all over the chicken.

Cook the chicken in oil thoroughly, for 5 minutes on each side, and then slice the chicken pieces into ½-inch slices.

Boil the pasta in the water. When it is cooked, drain the pasta and mix in the butter while the noodles are still hot.

Assemble the dish by covering the pasta in sauce, placing the bean mixture over it, and then adding the chicken. Garnish the dish by topping everything with the tomatoes and green onions.

Nutrition: Calories: 966, Fat: 18 g, Carbs: 34 g, Protein: 0 g, Sodium: 0 g

Olive Garden's Chicken Marsala

Preparation Time: 10 minutes

Cooking Time: 40 minutes

Servings: 6

Ingredients:

2 tablespoons olive oil

2 tablespoons butter

4 boneless skinless chicken breasts

1 ½ cups sliced mushrooms

1 small clove garlic, thinly sliced

Flour for dredging

Sea salt and freshly ground black pepper

1 ½ cups chicken stock

1 ½ cups Marsala wine

1 tablespoon lemon juice

1 teaspoon Dijon mustard

Directions:

Chicken scaloppini

Pound out the chicken with a mallet or rolling pin to about ½ inch thick

In a large skillet, heat the olive oil and 1 tablespoon of the butter over medium-high heat. When the oil is hot, dredge the chicken in flour. Season with salt and pepper on both sides. Dredge only as many as will fit in the skillet. Don't overcrowd the pan.

Cook chicken in batches, about 1 to 2 minutes on each side or until cooked through. Remove from skillet, and place on an oven-proof platter. Keep warm, in oven, while remaining chicken is cooked.

Marsala sauce

In the same skillet, add 1 tablespoon of olive oil. On medium-high heat, sauté mushrooms and garlic until softened. Remove the mushrooms from the pan and set aside.

Add the chicken stock and loosen any remaining bits in the pan. On high heat, let reduce by half, about 6-8 minutes. Add Marsala wine and lemon juice and in the same manner reduce by half, about 6–8 minutes. Add the mushroom back in the saucepan, and stir in the Dijon mustard. Warm for 1 minute on medium-low heat. Remove from heat, stir in the remaining butter to make the sauce silkier.

To serve, pour sauce over chicken, and serve immediately.

Nutrition: Calories: 950, Fat: 58 g, Carbs: 71 g, Protein: 66 g, Sodium: 1910 mg

Chili's Crispy Honey-Chipotle Chicken Crispers

Preparation Time: 15 minutes

Cooking Time: 30 minutes

Servings: 4

Ingredients:

Chicken: 12 chicken tenderloins

Some shortening or 6 cups vegetable oil for frying

Honey-Chipotle Sauce:

⅔ cup honey

¼ cup water

¼ cup ketchup

1 tablespoon white vinegar

2 teaspoons chipotle chili pepper, ground or powdered

½ teaspoon salt

Batter:

1 egg, beaten

½ cup whole milk

½ cup chicken broth

1½ teaspoons salt

¼ teaspoon black pepper

¼ teaspoon paprika

¼ teaspoon garlic powder

¾ cup all-purpose flour

Breading:

1½ cups all-purpose flour

1½ teaspoons salt

¾ teaspoon paprika

½ teaspoon black pepper

½ teaspoon garlic powder

Garnish:

French fries

Corn on the cub

Ranch dipping sauce

Directions:

Mix together all the chipotle sauce ingredients in a saucepan and bring to a boil over medium heat. When the sauce starts boiling, reduce it to a simmer and leave it for another two minutes before removing from heat.

Preheat the oil to 350°F. While you are waiting for your oil to heat, whisk all the batter ingredients (except the flour) together for 30 seconds, or until thoroughly mixed. When everything is mixed, add in the flour and mix again.

Add all the breading ingredients to another bowl.

Place the batter and breading bowls beside each other to make your coating station. The oil should be hot enough now.

Dip the chicken into the batter, let the excess batter drip off, and then dip it in the breading to coat.

Place the breaded chicken on a plate and start frying, two at a time at most. Leave each chicken piece in the oil for at least 4 minutes.

Prepare a plate by covering it with paper towels.

When the chicken is done cooking, transfer it to the paper towels to let the oil drain off.

Let the fried chicken cool, and then transfer it to a deep bowl. Add in the sauce and toss everything together. Make sure you cover the chicken in sauce.

Transfer to a plate and serve with sides of French fries, corn on the cub, and ranch dipping sauce.

Nutrition: Calories: 492, Fat: 3.3 g, Carbs: 107.2 g, Protein: 11.2 g, Sodium: 2331.5 mg

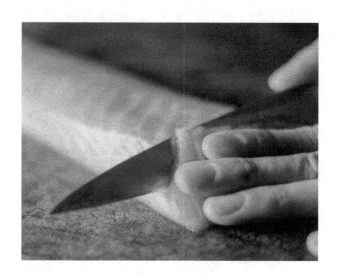

__Lunch (Fish)__

Applebee's Honey Grilled Salmon

Preparation Time: 10 minutes

Cooking Time: 30 minutes

Servings: 4

Ingredients:

Honey Pepper Sauce:

¾ cup honey

⅓ cup soy sauce

¼ cup dark brown sugar, packed

¼ cup pineapple juice

2 tablespoons fresh lemon juice

2 tablespoons white distilled vinegar

2 teaspoons olive oil

1 teaspoon black pepper, ground

½ teaspoon cayenne pepper

½ teaspoon paprika

¼ teaspoon garlic powder

Fish:

4 salmon fillets, 8 ounces each, skinned

Directions:

Cook all of the sauce ingredients over medium to low heat until boiling. Once the mixture boils, lower the heat a little and allow it to simmer for another 15 minutes.

Rub the salmon with vegetable oil, salt, and pepper, and grill for 4 to 7 minutes on each side.

Serve with the honey pepper sauce.

Nutrition: Calories: 579.6, Fat: 12.3 g, Carbs: 70.5 g, Protein: 49 g, Sodium: 1515.1 mg

Red Lobster's Maple-Glazed Salmon and Shrimp

Preparation Time: 10 minutes

Cooking Time: 20 minutes

Servings: 4

Ingredients:

⅔ cup maple syrup

½ cup water

2 tablespoons dried cherries, minced

1 tablespoon sugar

2 teaspoons soy sauce

1½ teaspoons lemon juice

24 pieces fresh medium shrimp, peeled

24 ounces salmon fillets

Directions:

To get started:

a)   Skewer the shrimp on 4 skewers (i.e. 6 shrimp each);

b)   Season the shrimp with salt and pepper; and

c)   Season the salmon with salt and pepper.

Combine the maple syrup, water, cherries, sugar soy sauce and lemon juice and bring to a boil over medium heat. Reduce the heat and allow the mixture to simmer for another 8 to 10 minutes.

Grill the shrimp over high heat for 1 to 2 minutes per side. When you're done with the shrimp, grill the salmon over high heat for 3 to 4 minutes per side.

Arrange the shrimp and salmon on a plate and serve with the maple sauce.

Nutrition: Calories: 364.7, Fat: 7.4 g, Carbs: 38.7 g, Protein: 34.8 g, Sodium: 301.1 mg

Chili's Garlic and Lime Shrimp

Preparation Time: 5 minutes

Cooking Time: 20 minutes

Servings: 4

Ingredients:

Shrimp:

2 tablespoons butter

1 clove garlic, chopped

32 fresh medium shrimp, peeled

1 lime, halved

Seasoning:

¾ teaspoon salt

¼ teaspoon ground black pepper

¼ teaspoon cayenne pepper

¼ teaspoon dried parsley flakes

¼ teaspoon garlic powder

¼ teaspoon paprika

⅛ teaspoon dried thyme

⅛ teaspoon onion powder

Directions:

Stir all the seasoning ingredients together to make the seasoning mix.

Sauté the garlic in the butter over medium heat for a few seconds before adding the shrimp to the pan. Squeeze the lime over the shrimp and continue to sauté it.

Stir in the seasoning mix, and continue sautéing the mixture for another 5 to 8 minutes.

Transfer to a plate and serve with thin lime wedges.

Nutrition: Calories: 89.1, Fat: 6.3 g, Carbs: 2.9 g, Protein: 6 g, Sodium: 725.4 mg

Red Lobster's Nantucket Baked Cod

Preparation Time: 10 minutes

Cooking Time: 30 minutes

Servings: 4

Ingredients:

Fish:

4 fresh cod fish fillets, about 1 ½ pounds in total

1 tablespoon butter, melted

½ lemon, juiced

2 small tomatoes, sliced

2 tablespoons grated parmesan cheese

Spice Blend:

¼ teaspoon salt

¼ teaspoon paprika

1 dash black pepper

1 dash cayenne pepper

Directions:

To get started:

a) Preheat the oven to 450°F; and

b) Prepare a 9×13 baking pan.

Place all the ingredients for the spice blend in a bowl and mix thoroughly.

Place the cod filets in the baking pan and brush with the tops with the butter.

Sprinkle the lemon juice and spice blend over the filets until you have finished all the spice blend.

Place 2 to 3 tomato slices on top of the spices for each fish.

Cover each slice of tomato with parmesan cheese.

Bake the fish for 8 minutes, then broil it on high for another 6 to 8 minutes.

Transfer the fish to a serving dish and serve with rice.

Nutrition: Calories: 187.9, Fat: 4.9 g, Carbs: 2.8 g, Protein: 31.9 g, Sodium: 303.6 mg

Chili's Crunchy Fried Shrimp

Preparation Time: 10 minutes

Cooking Time: 1 minute

Servings: 8

Ingredients:

2 pounds large shrimp, peeled

Crisco shortening, melted

Corn flake crumbs

Batter:

⅔ cup flour

1⅓ cups cornstarch

½ teaspoon salt

½ teaspoon baking powder

6 egg whites

⅔ cup water

4 tablespoons vegetable oil

Directions:

Mix the batter ingredients together and set aside.

In a separate container, pour out the cornflake crumbs.

Preheat the oil over medium heat.

Coat each shrimp with a generous amount of batter and then roll it in the crumbs.

Deep fry the shrimp until golden brown.

Place the shrimp on oil absorbent paper or paper towels.

Serve with cocktail or tartar sauce.

Nutrition: Calories: 272.9, Fat: 8.1 g, Carbs: 28.7 g, Protein: 19.3 g, Sodium: 854.2 mg

Applebee's Garlic and Peppercorn Fried Shrimp

Preparation Time:5 minutes

Cooking Time: 30 minutes

Servings: 4

Ingredients:

Shrimp:

1 pound shrimp, peeled, deveined, and tail removed

Vegetable oil, as needed

Flour Mixture:

½ cup wheat flour

¼ teaspoon salt

1 teaspoon ground black pepper

1 teaspoon granulated garlic

½ teaspoon paprika

1 teaspoon granulated sugar

Eggs:

2 eggs, beaten

Breading:

1 cup breadcrumbs

1 teaspoon ground black pepper

Directions:

Heat 3 inches of oil to 350°F.

Place the ingredients for the flour mixture in a bowl and mix. In separate bowls, beat the eggs and mix the breading ingredients together.

Dip the eggs in the flour mixture, then the eggs, then the breading.

After dipping, place the shrimp directly into the heated oil and cook for 2 to 3 minutes.

Place the cooked shrimp on a serving plate and serve with ketchup or tartar sauce.

Nutrition: Calories: 284.4, Fat: 5.4 g, Carbs: 34 g, Protein: 24.4 g , Sodium: 1021.5 mg

Cheesecake Factory's Bang Bang Chicken and Shrimp

Preparation Time: 10 minutes

Cooking Time: 50 minutes

Servings: 4

Ingredients:

Curry Sauce:

2 teaspoons chili oil

¼ cup onion

2 tablespoons garlic cloves, minced

2 teaspoons ginger

1 cup chicken broth

½ teaspoon cumin, ground

½ teaspoon coriander, ground

½ teaspoon paprika

¼ teaspoon salt

¼ teaspoon black pepper, ground

¼ teaspoon mace, ground

¼ teaspoon turmeric

3 cups coconut milk

2 medium carrots, julienned

1 small zucchini, julienned

½ cup peas, frozen

Peanut Sauce:

¼ cup creamy peanut butter

2 tablespoons water

4 teaspoons sugar

1 tablespoon soy sauce

1 teaspoon rice vinegar

1 teaspoon lime juice

½ teaspoon chili oil

Protein:

2 chicken breast fillets, cut into bite-sized pieces

16 large shrimp, raw, shelled

¼ cup cornstarch

½ cup vegetable oil

Final Dish:

1½ cups flaked coconut

4 cups white rice, cooked

½ teaspoon dried parsley, crumbled

2 tablespoons peanuts, finely chopped

2 green onions, julienned

Directions:

Sauté the onion, garlic, and ginger in heated chili oil for 30 seconds before adding in the broth.

Cook the mixture for another 30 seconds and then add in the cumin, coriander, paprika, salt, pepper, mace and turmeric.

Stir everything together and bring to a simmer. Keep the mixture at a simmer for 5 minutes and then add the coconut milk.

After adding the coconut milk, bring the mixture to a boil for 20 seconds.

Reduce the heat and then allow the mixture to simmer for 20 minutes before adding the carrots, zucchini, and peas.

Simmer the entire mixture for another 20 minutes and set the curry sauce aside. While waiting for the mixture to thicken, preheat the oven to 300°F.

Next, prepare the peanut sauce by mixing all of the ingredients together over medium heat.

When the peanut sauce starts to bubble, cover the pot, remove from heat, and set aside.

Spread the flaked coconut on a baking pan and bake for 30 minutes to toast. Swirl the flakes every 10 minutes, making sure they do not burn.

Pour the cornstarch in a bowl. Place the prepared chicken and shrimp into the bowl and cover entirely.

Sauté the chicken in the vegetable oil until it is cooked. Add the shrimp to the chicken and continue cooking.

Transfer the protein to a plate and set aside.

Arrange the dish as follows:

a)   Place some rice in the center of a plate;

b)   Place the chicken and shrimp around the rice;

c)   Pour the curry sauce over the chicken and the shrimp;

d)   Drizzle the peanut sauce over everything—especially the rice;

e)   Sprinkle some parsley and peanuts over the top of the rice, then top with the onions; then

f)   Sprinkle the toasted coconut flakes over the dish.

Serve and enjoy.

Nutrition: Calories: 1211, Fat: 84.2 g, Carbs: 101 g, Protein: 30 g, Sodium: 1940 mg

Disney World's Fulton's Crab House's Dungeness Crab Cakes

Preparation Time: 15 minutes

Cooking Time: 40 minutes

Servings: 4

Ingredients:

2½ pounds Dungeness crabmeat

1⅛ cups unsalted soda crackers, crushed

⅛ cup Dijon mustard

½ teaspoon Old Bay Seasoning

⅛ cup mayonnaise

1 egg

3 tablespoons butter, melted

1-2 lemon, cut into thin wedges for serving

Bearnaise sauce for serving, if desired

Directions:

To get started:

a) Squeeze the crab meat to remove moisture;

b) Preheat the oven to 425°F; and

c) Butter a baking sheet.

Mix the mustard, seasoning, mayonnaise, and egg in a bowl. Refrigerate for 10 minutes.

Remove the mixture from the refrigerator, and add in the cracker crumbs. Continue mixing.

Pour the mixture over the crab and continue mixing.

Divide the mixture into 12, and then shape each dollop into a 1-inch thick circle.

Place the cakes on the baking sheet and drizzle some butter over each.

Bake for 15 to 20 minutes, until cakes are cooked through. Serve with lemon wedges and béarnaise sauce, if desired.

Nutrition: Calories: 200, Fat: 6 g, Carbs: 18 g, Protein: 18 g, Sodium: 502 mg

Olive Garden's Chicken and Shrimp Carbonara

Preparation Time: 35 minutes

Cooking Time: 40 minutes

Servings: 8

Ingredients:

Shrimp Marinade

¼ cup extra virgin olive oil

½ cup water

2 teaspoons Italian seasoning

1 tablespoon minced garlic

Chicken:

4 boneless and skinless chicken breasts cubed

1 egg mixed with 1 tablespoon cold water

½ cup panko bread crumbs

½ cup all-purpose flour

½ teaspoon salt

½ teaspoon black pepper

2 tablespoons olive oil

Carbonara sauce:

½ cup butter (1 stick)

3 tablespoons all-purpose flour

½ cup parmesan cheese, grated

2 cups heavy cream

2 cups milk

8 Canadian bacon slices, diced finely

¾ cup roasted red peppers, diced

Pasta:

1 teaspoon salt

14 ounces spaghetti or bucatini pasta (1 package)

Water to cook the pasta

Shrimp:

½ pound fresh medium shrimp, deveined and peeled

1-2 tablespoons olive oil for cooking

Directions:

Mix all the marinade ingredients together in a re-sealable container or bag and add the add shrimp. Refrigerate for at least 30 minutes.

To make the chicken: Mix the flour, salt, pepper, and panko bread crumbs into a shallow dish. Whisk the egg with 1 tablespoon of cold water in a second shallow dish. Dip the chicken into the breadcrumb mix and after in the egg wash, and again in the breadcrumb mix. Place on a plate and let rest until all the chicken is prepared.

Warm the olive oil over medium heat in a deep large skillet. Working in batches, add the chicken. Cook for 4 to 6 minutes per side or until the chicken is cooked through. Place the cooked chicken tenders on a plate lined with paper towels to absorb excess oil.

To make the pasta: Add water to large pot and bring to a boil. Add salt and cook the pasta according to package instructions about 10-15 minutes before the sauce is ready.

To make the shrimp: While the pasta is cooking, add olive oil to a skillet. Remove the shrimp from the marinate and shake off the excess marinade. Cook the shrimp until they turn pink, about 2-3 minutes.

To make the Carbonara sauce: in a large deep skillet, sauté the Canadian bacon with a bit of butter for 3-4 minutes over medium heat or until the bacon starts to caramelize. Add the garlic and sauté for 1 more minute. Remove bacon and garlic and set aside.

In the same skillet, let the butter melt and mix-in the flour. Gradually add the cream and milk and whisk until the sauce thickens. Add the cheese.

Reduce the heat to a simmer and keep the mixture simmering while you prepare the rest of the ingredients.

When you are ready to serve, add the drained pasta, bacon bits, roasted red peppers to sauce. Stir to coat. Add pasta evenly to each serving

plate. Top with some chicken and shrimp. Garnish with fresh parsley
Serve with fresh shredded Romano or Parmesan cheese

Nutrition: Calories: 1570, Fat: 113 g, Carbs: 84 g, Protein: 55 g, Sodium: 2400 mg

Bubba Gump Shrimp Company's Cajun Shrimp

Preparation Time: 5 minutes

Cooking Time: 15 minutes

Servings: 4

Ingredients:

2 teaspoons paprika

1 teaspoon dried thyme

½ teaspoon salt

¼ teaspoon nutmeg, ground

¼ teaspoon garlic powder

⅛ teaspoon cayenne pepper

1 tablespoon olive oil

1 pound fresh medium-sized shrimp, peeled, deveined

Directions:

Sauté all the ingredients (except for the shrimp) in oil for 30 seconds.

When the ingredients have heated up, add the shrimp and continue sautéing for 2 to 3 minutes.

When the shrimp is cooked entirely, transfer to a plate and serve.

Nutrition: Calories: 270, Fat: 234 g, Carbs: 169 g, Protein: 70 g, Sodium: 2878 mg

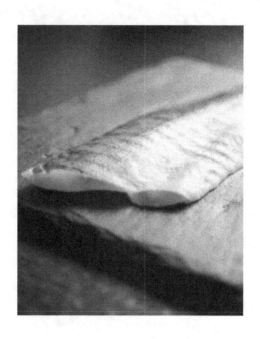

Herb Grilled Salmon

Preparation Time: 10 minutes

Cooking Time: 10 minutes

Servings: 4

Ingredients:

4 salmon steaks

Olive oil for brushing

Salt and pepper to taste

Lemon herb butter:

1 pound butter

1½ lemons (zest and juice but no seeds)

1 tablespoon fresh chopped herbs like basil and thyme

2 teaspoons fresh parsley, chopped

Directions:

To make the lemon herb butter, combine the butter, lemon zest, lemon juice and herbs in a food processor. Blend until smooth. Transfer to plastic wrap. Shape into a log and twist to seal. Chill in the refrigerator for up to three weeks.

Preheat a gas grill on medium heat or start a medium fire in a charcoal grill.

Brush the olive oil onto the fish fillets. Sprinkle with salt and pepper. Grill until fully cooked (when the salmon begins to change colors and becomes flaky).

Remove from the grill and top with the lemon herb butter. Serve.

Nutrition: Calories: 122, Fat: 23 g, Carbs: 33 g, Protein: 24 g, Sodium: 428 mg

Fettuccine with Shrimp and Zucchini

Preparation Time: 10 minutes

Cooking Time: 7 minutes

Servings: 4

Ingredients:

1 pound dry fettuccine

½ cup extra-virgin olive oil

1 tablespoon garlic, chopped

2 tablespoons parsley, chopped

1 medium zucchini

1 pound large shrimp

1 cup dry white wine

¾ teaspoon salt

¾ teaspoon black pepper

¼ cup butter

6 lemon wedges

1 sprig parsley, chopped

Directions:

Slice zucchini into approximately 2×¼-inch sticks. Peel and devein shrimp.

Cook pasta according to package directions. Drain and set aside.

In a sauté pan, heat the oil over medium heat. Cook garlic and parsley for 1 minute.

Add the zucchini slices and cook for 1 minute. Add the shrimp, wine, salt, pepper, and butter. Stir and cook the shrimp for 5 minutes.

Toss the pasta into the saucepan. Mix well. Squeeze some lemon over the pasta. Serve.

Nutrition: Calories: 153, Fat: 24.5 g, Carbs: 16. 5 g, Protein: 35 g, Sodium: 645 mg

<u>Dinner</u>

Make-At-Home KFC Original Fried Chicken

Preparation Time: 20 minutes

Cooking Time: 40 minutes

Servings: 4

Ingredients:

Spice mix:

1 tablespoon paprika

2 teaspoons onion salt

1 teaspoon chili powder

1 teaspoon black pepper, ground

½ teaspoon celery salt

½ teaspoon dried sage

½ teaspoon garlic powder

½ teaspoon allspice, ground

½ teaspoon dried oregano

½ teaspoon dried basil

½ teaspoon dried marjoram

Chicken preparation:

1 whole chicken, cut into parts

2 quarts frying oil

1 egg white

1 ½ cups all-purpose flour

1 tablespoon brown sugar

1 tablespoon kosher salt

Directions:

Preheat oil in deep-fryer to 350°F.

In a bowl, mix together ingredients for the spice mix. Then, add flour, sugar, and salt. Mix well until fully blended.

Coat each chicken piece with egg white, then the flour breading. Make sure that the chicken pieces are well-coated.

Transfer to a plate and allow chicken to dry for about 5 minutes.

Deep-fry breasts and wings together for about 12 minutes or until the temperature on a meat thermometer inserted in the breast's thickest part reads 165 °F. Do the same with legs and thighs. Usually these parts take 1-2 minutes more to cook.

Transfer pieces onto a plate lined with paper towels.

Serve.

Nutrition: Calories 418 Total, Fat 22 g, Carbs 41 g, Protein 15 g, Sodium 1495 mg

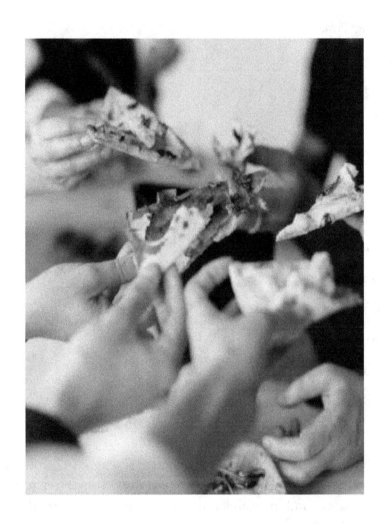

Copycat California Pizza Kitchen's California Club Pizza

Preparation Time: 5 minutes

Cooking Time: 12 minutes

Servings: 4

Ingredients:

1 ball pizza dough

2 tablespoons olive oil

1 chicken breast, cooked and chopped into bite-sized pieces

4 slices of bacon, cooked and cut into bite-sized pieces

1 cup mozzarella cheese, grated

1½ cups arugula

2 tablespoons mayonnaise

1 tomato, sliced

1 avocado, peeled and cut into 8 slices

Directions:

Preheat pizza stone in oven to 425°F.

Using a rolling pin, flatten pizza dough until it is about 12 to 14 inches in diameter. Brush olive oil in a thin and even layer on top. Add chicken, bacon, and mozzarella in layers evenly across pizza dough.

Place onto pizza stone and bake for about 10 to 12 minutes or until cheese melts and crust is slightly brown. Remove from oven and set aside.

In a bowl, add arugula and mayonnaise. Mix well. Top cooked pizza with tomato, arugula mixture, and avocado.

Serve warm.

Nutrition: Calories 456, Total fat 32 g, Saturated fat 8 g, Carbs 18 g, Sugar 2 g, Fibers 4 g, Protein 26 g, Sodium 625 mg

Oriental Salad from Applebee's

Preparation Time: 15 minutes

Cooking Time: 5 minutes

Servings: 6

Ingredients:

3 tablespoons honey

1½ tablespoons rice wine vinegar

¼ cup mayonnaise

1 teaspoon Dijon mustard

⅛ teaspoon sesame oil

3 cups vegetable oil, for frying

2 chicken breasts, cut into thin strips

1 egg

1 cup milk

1 cup flour

1 cup breadcrumbs

1 teaspoon salt

¼ teaspoon pepper

3 cups romaine lettuce, diced

½ cup red cabbage, diced

½ cup napa cabbage, diced

1 carrot, grated

¼ cup cucumber, diced

3 tablespoons sliced almonds

¼ cup dry chow mein

Directions:

To make the dressing, add honey, rice wine vinegar, mayonnaise, Dijon mustard, and sesame oil to a blender. Mix until well combined. Store in refrigerator until ready to serve.

Heat oil in a deep pan over medium-high heat.

As oil warms, whisk together egg and milk in a bowl. In another bowl, add flour, breadcrumbs, salt, and pepper. Mix well.

Dredge chicken strips in egg mixture, then in the flour mixture. Make sure the chicken is coated evenly on all sides. Shake off any excess.

Deep fry chicken strips for about 3 to 4 minutes until thoroughly cooked and lightly brown. Transfer onto a plate lined with paper towels to drain and cool. Work in batches, if necessary.

Chop strips into small, bite-size pieces once cool enough to handle.

Next, prepare salad by adding romaine, red cabbage, napa cabbage, carrots, and cucumber to a serving bowl. Top with chicken pieces, almonds, and chow mein. Drizzle prepared dressing on top.

Serve immediately.

Nutrition: Calories 384, Total fat 13 g, Saturated fat 3 g, Carbs 40 g, Sugar 13 g, Fibers 2 g, Protein 27 g, Sodium 568 mg

Other Restaurant Favorites I

Chick-fil-A Chicken Nuggets with Honey Mustard Dipping Sauce

Preparation Time: 15 minutes

Cooking Time: 15 minutes

Servings: 4

Ingredients:

1 egg

¾ cup milk

¼ cup dill pickle juice

2 large chicken breasts, cut into bite-sized pieces

Salt and pepper to taste

1¼ cups all-purpose flour

2 tablespoons powdered sugar

2 teaspoons salt

1 teaspoon pepper

½ cup canola oil

½ cup plain Greek yogurt

1½ tablespoons yellow mustard

1 tablespoon Dijon mustard

2 tablespoons honey

Directions:

Mix egg, milk, and pickle juice in a bowl until well combined. Season chicken pieces with salt and pepper and then add to egg mixture. Refrigerate for at least 2 hours to marinate.

In another bowl, add flour, powdered sugar, salt, and pepper. Mix well until combined. Transfer chicken from marinade into flour mixture. Toss and fold to coat thoroughly and evenly on all sides.

Heat ½ cup oil in a large pan over medium-high heat. The oil is hot enough if it sizzles when you sprinkle a little of the flour mixture on top but if it pops, it's too hot. Lower temperature if this happens.

One at a time, slowly add chicken into hot oil. Allow spacing between pieces. Deep fry pieces for about 3 to 4 minutes until one side is lightly brown. Using tongs, turn pieces over and continue cooking for another 3 to 4 minutes. Transfer to a plate lined with paper towels.

To make the dipping sauce, combine Greek yogurt, both mustards, and honey in a bowl. Mix well. Serve on the side with hot chicken pieces.

Nutrition: Calories 395, Total fat 6 g, Saturated fat 2 g, Carbs 45 g, Sugar 16 g, Fibers 2 g, Protein 39 g, Sodium 1434 mg

Red Lobster's Garlic Shrimp Scampi

Preparation Time: 15 minutes

Cooking Time: 15 minutes

Servings: 4

Ingredients:

1 pound shrimp, peeled and deveined

Salt and pepper to taste

1 tablespoon olive oil

3 garlic cloves, finely chopped

1½ white wine

2 tablespoons lemon juice

¼ teaspoon dried basil

¼ teaspoon dried oregano

¼ teaspoon dried rosemary

¼ teaspoon dried thyme

½ cup butter

2 tablespoons parsley leaves, minced

¼ cup Parmesan cheese, shredded (optional)

Directions:

Flavor shrimp with salt and pepper.

In a pan with heated oil, sauté shrimp on medium-high heat for about 2 minutes or until color changes to pink. Transfer onto a plate for later.

In the same pan, sauté garlic for 30 seconds or until aromatic. Pour in white wine and lemon juice. Stir, then bring to a boil. Adjust heat to medium-low and cook for an additional 4 minutes. Mix in basil, oregano, rosemary, and thyme. Then, add butter gradually. Mix until completely melted and blended with other ingredients. Remove from heat.

Return shrimp to pan and add parsley. Taste and adjust seasoning with salt and pepper as needed.

Sprinkle Parmesan on top, if desired. Serve.

Nutrition: Calories 448, Total Fat 29 g, Carbs 3 g, Protein 26 g, Sodium 362 mg

121

Bonefish Grill's Bang Bang Shrimp

Preparation Time: 5 minutes

Cooking Time: 5 minutes

Servings: 4

Ingredients:

½ cup mayonnaise

¼ cup Thai sweet chili sauce

3-5 drops hot chili sauce (or more if you like it spicier)

½ cup cornstarch

1 pound small shrimp, peeled and deveined

1½ cups vegetable oil

Directions:

To make the sauce, combine mayonnaise with Thai chili sauce and hot chili sauce in a bowl.

In a separate bowl, add cornstarch. Toss shrimp in cornstarch until well-coated.

Heat oil in a wok. Working in batches, fry shrimp until golden brown, about 2-3 minutes. Transfer onto a plate lined with paper towels to drain excess oil.

Serve shrimp in a bowl with sauce drizzled on top.

Nutrition: Calories 274, Total Fat 11 g, Carbs 26 g, Protein 16 g, Sodium 1086 mg

Chi-Chi's Seafood Chimichanga

Preparation Time: 10 minutes

Cooking Time: 30 minutes

Servings: 6

Ingredients:

4 tablespoons butter

4 tablespoons flour

½ teaspoon butter

2 dashes black pepper, ground

2 cups milk

8 ounces jack cheese, shredded

1 16-ounce package crab meat, flaked

1 cup cottage cheese

¼ cup Parmesan cheese

1 egg

1 tablespoon dried parsley flakes

¼ teaspoon onion powder

1 tablespoon lemon juice

Shredded lettuce for serving

¼ cup sliced green onions for garnish

Directions:

Preheat oven to 375°F.

To make the sauce, heat butter in a pan on medium heat. Add flour, salt, and pepper. Mix, then pour in milk. Stirring often, cook until sauce is thick then simmer for an additional 1 minute.

Turn off heat and stir in jack cheese until completely blended into sauce.

In a bowl, combine crab meat, cottage and Parmesan cheese, egg, parsley, and onion powder. Heat tortillas in microwave for 10 seconds or until warm. Wet bottom side of tortilla and add crab meat mixture on top. Fold tortilla to wrap filling.

Coat baking sheet with cooking spray. Bake chimichangas for about 25 minutes.

Reheat sauce until warm. Mix in lemon juice and stir until blended.

Transfer chimichangas to plates over a bed of shredded lettuce, if desired. Top with sauce and garnish with green onions before serving.

Nutrition: Calories 794, Total Fat 33 g, Carbs 77 g, Protein 44 g, Sodium 1932 mg

Red Lobster's Copycat Lobster Pizza

Preparation Time: 15 minutes

Cooking Time: 5 minutes

Servings: 1

Ingredients:

1 10-inch flour tortillas

1 ounce roasted garlic butter

2 tablespoons Parmesan cheese, shredded

1/2 cup fresh Roma tomatoes, finely chopped

2 tablespoons fresh basil, cut into thin strips

2 ounces lobster meat, chopped

½ cup Italian cheese blend, grated

Vegetable oil for coating

Dash salt and pepper

Fresh lemon juice for serving

Directions:

Preheat oven to 450°F.

Coat one side of tortilla with garlic butter. Top with Parmesan cheese, tomatoes, basil, lobster meat, and Italian cheese blend in that order. Set aside.

Prepare a pizza pan. Apply a light coat of vegetable oil and cover with a dash of salt and pepper. Transfer pizza onto pan. Bake for about 5 minutes.

Cut into slices and drizzle with lemon juice.

Serve.

Nutrition: Calories 339, Total Fat 10 g, Carbs 41 g, Protein 22 g, Sodium 890 mg

Bonefish Grill's Skewered Shrimp with Pan-Asian Glaze

Preparation Time: 5 minutes

Cooking Time: 10 minutes

Servings: 4

Ingredients:

¼ ketchup

¼ cup oyster sauce

1 tablespoon soy sauce

1 tablespoon water

¾ tablespoon lemon juice

1 tablespoon extra-virgin olive oil, plus more

1 tablespoon fresh ginger, peeled and finely chopped

1 tablespoon sugar

1 tablespoon honey

1 pound shrimp, peeled, deveined, and skewered

Preparation:

In a bowl, add ketchup, oyster sauce, soy sauce, water, and lemon juice. Mix well.

Add olive oil to a deep pan over medium heat. Once hot, stir fry ginger for about 1 minute until aromatic. Pour in ketchup mixture. Once simmering, lower heat to medium-low. Add sugar and honey. Cook for 1 minute, stirring frequently. Remove from heat. Set aside.

Preheat grill over high heat. Coat top with olive oil. Dry shrimp with a paper towel, then season all sides with salt and pepper. Add to grill and cook for 1 to 2 minutes until color changes. Turn shrimp, then coat cooked side with prepared glaze mixture. Grill until bottom side is cooked, then turn again. Apply glaze to other side. Remove from grill.

Serve.

Nutrition: Calories 199, Total fat 5 g, Saturated fat 1 g, Carbs 14 g, Sugar 8 g, Fibers 0 g, Protein 24 g, Sodium 750 mg

DIY Red Hook's Lobster Pound

Preparation Time: 10 minutes

Cooking Time: 10 minutes

Servings: 2

Ingredients:

2 large egg yolks

1 teaspoon Dijon mustard

4 teaspoons fresh lemon juice, plus more

1 cup vegetable oil

Coarse salt and ground pepper, to taste

¾ pounds lobster meat, cooked and chopped into 1-inch cubes

2 top-split hot dog rolls

2 tablespoons butter, melted

Iceberg lettuce, shredded

1 scallion, finely sliced

Paprika, to taste

Directions:

To make the DIY mayonnaise, add egg yolks, mustard, and lemon juice to a food processor. Process until fully mixed. Then, while still processing, gradually add oil until mixture thickens and becomes cloudy. Add salt and pepper.

Transfer to a bowl and cover. Set aside.

Prepare lobster filling by combining lobster pieces, prepared mayonnaise, lemon juice, salt, and pepper in a bowl.

Heat griddle. Apply butter to insides of hotdog rolls. Place rolls to grill butter side down, and cook until golden brown.

Assemble lobster rolls by layering lettuce, lobster and mayonnaise mixture, scallions, and paprika. Repeat for 2nd lobster roll.

Serve.

Nutrition: Calories 1746, Total fat 135 g, Saturated fat 90 g, Carbs 49 g, Sugar 9 g, Fibers 5 g, Protein 92 g, Sodium 2299 mg

Copycat Bubba Gum's Coconut Shrimp

Preparation Time: 5 minutes

Cooking Time: 20 minutes

Servings: 2

Ingredients:

Oil, for deep frying

½ pound medium raw shrimp, peeled and deveined

¾ cup pancake mix

¾ cup wheat beer

¼ cup all-purpose flour

¼ teaspoon seasoning salt

¼ teaspoon cayenne pepper

¼ teaspoon garlic powder

1 cup shredded coconut

Sauce:

¼ cup orange marmalade

½ teaspoon Cajun seasoning

Directions:

Preheat deep fryer to 350°F.

Run cold water over shrimp then dry using a paper towel. Set aside.

Prepare 3 bowls for the different coatings. In the 1st bowl, combine pancake mix and beer. In the 2nd, combine flour, seasoning salt, cayenne pepper, and garlic powder. For the 3rd bowl, add coconut.

One at a time, dredge shrimp into 1st bowl, shaking excess flour, then into the 2nd bowl followed by the 3rd.

Deep fry shrimp for about 45 to 60 seconds until lightly brown. Then, transfer onto a plate lined with paper towels to drain.

Prepare dipping sauce by combining sauce ingredients in a bowl.

Serve shrimp with dipping sauce on the side.

Nutrition: Calories 609, Total fat 15 g, Saturated fat 12 g, Carbs 84 g, Sugar 35 g, Fibers 6 g, Protein 32 g, Sodium 1555 mg

T.G.I. Friday's Black Bean Soup

Preparation Time: 10 minutes

Cooking Time: 1 hour 15 minutes

Servings: 6

Ingredients:

2 tablespoons vegetable oil

¾ cup white onion, diced

¾ cup celery, diced

½ cup carrot, diced

¼ cup green bell pepper, diced

2 tablespoons garlic, minced

4 15-ounce cans black beans, rinsed

4 cups chicken stock

2 tablespoons apple cider vinegar

2 teaspoons chili powder

½ teaspoon cayenne pepper

½ teaspoon cumin

½ teaspoon salt

¼ teaspoon hickory liquid smoke

Directions:

In a pan, sauté the onion, celery, carrot, bell pepper, and garlic in the heated oil for 15 minutes over low heat. Make sure to keep the vegetables from burning.

While the vegetables are cooking, strain and wash the black beans.

Add 3 cups of the washed beans and a cup of chicken stock to a food processor and purée until smooth.

When the onion mixture is cooked, add the rest of the ingredients (including the bean purée) to the pan.

Bring everything to a boil, then lower the heat and allow the mixture to simmer for another 50 to 60 minutes.

Transfer the soup to bowls and serve.

Nutrition: Calories 392.5, Total Fat 7.8 g, Carbs 59.3 g, Protein 23 g, Sodium 458.9 mg

Olive Garden's Minestrone Soup

Preparation Time: 5 minutes

Cooking Time: 40 minutes

Servings: 8

Ingredients:

3 tablespoons olive oil

½ cup green beans, sliced

¼ cup celery, diced

1 cup white onion diced)

1 zucchini, diced

4 teaspoons minced garlic

4 cups vegetable broth

1 can (15 ounces each) red kidney beans, drained

2 cans (15 ounces each) small white beans, drained

1 can (14 ounce) tomatoes, diced

1 carrot, peeled and diced

2 tablespoons fresh Italian parsley, chopped finely

1½ teaspoons dried oregano

1½ teaspoons salt

½ teaspoon ground black pepper

½ teaspoon dried basil

¼ teaspoon dried thyme

3 cups hot water

4 cups fresh baby spinach

½ cup small shell pasta

Shredded parmesan cheese for serving

Directions:

Chop and mince the ingredients as specified.

Sauté the green beans, celery, onion, zucchini, and garlic in olive oil in a soup pot until the onions become translucent.

Add in the rest of the ingredients, except the beans, pasta, and spinach leaves, and bring the mixture to a boil.

When the mixture is boiling, add in the beans, spinach and pasta. Reduce the heat and allow to simmer for another 20 minutes.

Ladle into a bowl, sprinkle with parmesan if desired, and serve.

Nutrition: Calories 353.5, Total Fat 6.3 g, Carbs 57.8 g, Protein 19.2 g, Sodium 471.7 mg

Panera Bread's Vegetarian Summer Corn Chowder

Preparation Time: 10 minutes

Cooking Time: 45 minutes

Servings: 6

Ingredients:

2 tablespoons olive oil

1 tablespoon unsalted butter

1 medium red onion, diced

3 tablespoons all-purpose flour

2 russet potatoes, diced

5 cups unsalted vegetable stock

½ cup red bell pepper, diced

½ cup green bell pepper, diced

4 cups whole corn kernels

¼ teaspoon black pepper, ground

1 cup half-and-half cream

Salt and pepper to taste

Chives, thinly sliced, for garnish

Bacon bits, for garnish

Directions:

Sauté the onion in butter and oil over low heat. When the onion becomes translucent, add in the flour and cook for another 5 minutes.

Dice the potatoes into quarter-inch cubes and add it to the simmering mixture. Add the broth, then turn the heat up and bring the mixture to a boil.

Reduce the heat to medium and continue simmering for 15 minutes.

Dice the bell peppers into quarter-inch cubes and add them to the mixture. Also add in the corn, pepper, cream, salt, and pepper, and allow the mixture to simmer for another 15 minutes.

Transfer the soup into a bowl and garnish with chives and bacon, if desired.

Nutrition: Calories 320, Total Fat 20 g, Carbs 34 g, Protein 5 g, Sodium 1310 mg

Hostess® Twinkies

Preparation Time: 15 minutes

Cooking Time: 55 minutes

Servings: 2

Ingredients:

For Cake:

7 egg whites

½ teaspoon tartar cream

2 cups flour

1 ½ cups sugar

1 tablespoon baking powder

7 egg yolks

½ cup vegetable oil

¾ cup cold water

2 teaspoons vanilla

½ teaspoon salt

For Filling:

6 tablespoons flour (rounded)

1 ½ cups Butter Flavor Crisco

1 ½ cups sugar

1 cup cold milk (scant)

2 teaspoons vanilla

Directions:

Preheat your oven to 350 F.

Mix flour with baking powder, sugar & salt in a large sized bowl; mix well. Make a well in the middle & add in the oil, vanilla, cold water & egg yolks. Using a large spoon, beat well until smooth; set aside.

Beat whites with cream of tartar until stiff peaks appear. Transfer on top of the egg yolk batter & fold in until combined.

Transfer to a 10x14" pan, ungreased & bake for 45 to 50 minutes. Let cool for couple of minutes and then turn upside down into another pan. Let cool, then run a knife around the edges. Remove & cut in half.

Now, for the filling, mix flour together with Butter Flavor Crisco & sugar; beat for 4 to 5 minutes on high & then gradually add in vanilla & milk. Beat on high again for 3 to 5 more minutes. Spread the mixture between 2 even layers & cut it into 3x1" size & wrap them individually

Nutrition: Calories: 3391 kcal, Protein: 41.21 g, Fat: 239.44 g, Carbohydrates: 273.27 g

Hostess® Sno Balls®

Preparation Time: 15 minutes

Cooking Time: 1 hour & 10 minutes

Servings: 10

Ingredients:

For the Cake:

3 eggs

1 stick butter, unsalted, softened

2 teaspoons baking soda

1 teaspoon of vanilla extract

2 cups all-purpose flour

1/3 cup cocoa powder

2 cups sugar

1 ½ cups milk

½ teaspoon salt

For the Frosting:

3 drops of red food coloring

1 ½ cups sugar

6 egg whites

1 teaspoon cream of tarter

2 cups coconut, shredded

1 teaspoon coconut extract

2 teaspoons vanilla extract

1/3 cup water

Directions:

For the Cake:

Cream butter with the sugar & then gradually add in vanilla & eggs. Whisk flour together with the cocoa, baking soda & salt in a separate large sized bowl.

Add half of the dry mixture to sugar/butter mixture & then add in the milk and the remaining dry mixture.

Scoop everything into a lightly greased muffin tin & bake for 15 minutes at 350 F. Allow it to cool for some time at room temperature.

Cut a cone from the bottom of every cake & trim the tip off.

For the Filling:

Beat the egg whites well until soft peaks form, for couple of minutes.

Combine sugar together with cream of tartar & water in a small sized saucepan; bring everything to a boil, over moderate heat settings. Remove the pan from heat & let cool a bit at room temperature.

Gradually pour the syrup into the egg whites and then add in vanilla & coconut extract.

Whip until the mixture is thickened, for 10 more minutes. Process the coconut in a food processor. If desired, feel free to add food coloring during this process.

Replace the cap of the cake; leaving it upside down for the frosting.

Generously coat the bottom & sides with a layer of frosting and then add in the coconut sprinkles.

Nutrition: Calories: 400 kcal, Protein: 9.56 g, Carbohydrates: 59.84 g

Other Restaurant Favorites II

Hostess® Cupcakes

Preparation Time: 15 minutes

Cooking Time: 1 hour 15 minutes

Servings: 10

Ingredients:

For Cupcakes:

1 ½ cups sugar

2 cups flour

¾ cup Dutch process cocoa

1 teaspoon of baking powder

1 ½ teaspoons of baking soda

½ teaspoon salt

2 eggs

1 cup oil

¾ cup buttermilk

1 teaspoon vanilla

¾ cup hot coffee

For Ganache:

¾ cup cream

7 ounces chocolate

For Filling:

4 tablespoons butter

1 cup powdered sugar

2 teaspoons vanilla

1 cup marshmallow crème

For Icing:

½ stick butter

1 cup powdered sugar

½ teaspoon vanilla

½ -1 tablespoon milk

Directions:

Preheat your oven to 350 F. Sift flour together with Dutch process cocoa, sugar, baking soda, baking powder & salt in a large sized bowl. Beat eggs together with oil, vanilla & buttermilk in a separate bowl, and then add the mixture into the dry ingredients. Beat in the warm coffee.

Pour the mixture into the lined muffin cups & fill them approximately 2/3 full; bake for 18 to 20 minutes at 350 F. Remove from oven & let cool a bit at room temperature. Beat all the filling ingredients together in a medium sized bowl. Fill a large sized piping bag. When you can easily handle the cupcakes, press their tip into the middle & squeeze one or two tablespoons of cream filling into the middle. Repeat the process for all the cupcakes.

Over medium heat settings in a large saucepan; heat the cream until the cream is hot & just begins to boil, stirring frequently. Transfer the cream immediately on top of the chocolate; whisk until smooth. Spread the slightly cooled but warm ganache on top of the filled cupcakes.

Whip all the icing ingredients together until smooth; if required, feel free to add more of milk. Fill a piping bag & pipe on the curls.

Nutrition: Calories: 609 kcal, Protein: 7.19 g, Fat: 33.47 g, Carbohydrates: 73.72 g

Starbucks® Iced Lemon Pound Cake

Preparation Time: 15 minutes

Cooking Time: 1 hour

Servings: 12

Ingredients:

For Cake:

6 tablespoons lemon juice, freshly squeezed

1 package lemon pudding mix, non-instant (4.3 ounce)

8 ounces sour cream

1 package yellow cake mix (18.25 ounce)

½ cup milk

4 eggs, large

½ cup vegetable oil

For Icing:

3 tablespoons lemon juice, freshly squeezed or more to taste

2 ½ cups confectioners' sugar

Directions:

Lightly grease two loaf pans & preheat your oven to 350 F in advance.

Now, mix cake mix together with eggs, oil, pudding mix, sour cream, 6 tablespoons of the lemon juice, and milk in a stand mixer; beat for couple of minutes & then transfer the mixture into already prepared greased loaf pans.

Bake for 45 to 50 minutes, until a toothpick should come out clean. Before removing the cake from pans, let cool in the pans for couple of minutes & then transfer on a wire rack to completely cool.

Now, whisk the icing ingredients together in a medium sized bowl until smooth, for couple of minutes; evenly spoon the mixture over the loaves & let set for half an hour, before you slice them into pieces.

Nutrition: Calories: 414 kcal, Protein: 3.98 g, Fat: 15.39 g, Carbohydrates: 66.83 g

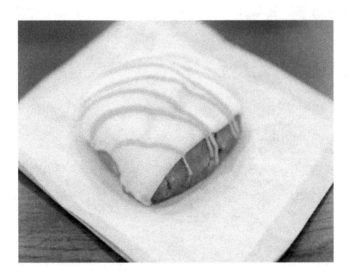

Starbucks® Banana Bread

Preparation Time: 15 minutes

Cooking Time: 50 minutes

Servings: 8

Ingredients:

3 ripe bananas, medium-large, mashed

1/3 cup chopped walnuts (in addition to 1/2 cup)

1 egg, large

2 cups flour

½ cup plus 1/3 cup walnuts, chopped

1 teaspoon baking soda

½ teaspoon vanilla extract

2 tablespoons buttermilk

½ cup vegetable oil

1 1/8 cups sugar

¼ teaspoon salt

Directions:

Lightly grease a 9x5x3" loaf pan with the oil, dust with the flour & then preheat your oven to 325 F.

Blend baking soda together with flour & salt; set aside. Now, mix egg with vegetable oil & sugar until combined well.

Gradually add flour mixture to the egg mixture; blend well & then, add in the mashed bananas, vanilla & buttermilk; mix well. Fold approximately ½ cup of the chopped walnuts & transfer the batter into already prepared loaf pan.

Top the batter with the leftover walnuts. Bake until a toothpick comes out clean, for 50 to 60 minutes.

Nutrition: Calories: 350 kcal, Protein: 4.96 g, Fat: 19.94 g, Carbohydrates: 39.37 g

Starbucks® Vanilla Bean Scone

Preparation Time: 25 minutes

Cooking Time: 15 minutes

Servings: 16

Ingredients:

For Scones:

½ cup sugar

2 teaspoon vanilla extract

½ cup butter, cold, cubed

2 ½ cup all-purpose flour

½ cup heavy cream

1 tablespoon baking powder

½ vanilla bean, scraped

1 egg, large

¼ teaspoon salt

For Glaze:

6-7 tablespoon Heavy Cream

½ Vanilla Bean, scraped

1 teaspoon Vanilla Extract

3 cups powdered sugar

Directions:

Line a large baking sheet either with a silicone mat or parchment paper & preheat your oven to 400 F in advance.

Combine flour together with baking powder, salt & sugar. Pulse in a food processor or whisk until evenly mixed.

Add butter & pulse in a food processor or cut in using a pastry cutter until the mixture looks like a cornmeal texture.

Whisk cream together with egg, vanilla extract & scraping in a separate bowl.

Add liquid to the flour mixture & stir well using your hands until the dough forms a ball or pulse in a food processor until just combined.

Place the dough onto a lightly floured surface & then briefly knead until the dough comes together; roll the dough out to approximately ½ inch thickness.

Make 8 squares or rectangles from the dough & then cut each one diagonally & then create 32 small scones on the other.

Place them onto already prepared large sized baking sheet & bake or until the edges start to get golden brown, for 10 to 12 minutes.

Transfer the cooked scones to a cooling rack & let completely cool.

In the meantime; whisk the glaze ingredients together in a large sized bowl, keep adding one tablespoon of the cream until you get your desired thickness. Dip the cooled scones in the glaze & then place them onto cooling rack again until harden.

Nutrition: Calories: 247 kcal, Protein: 2.45 g, Fat: 9.87 g, Carbohydrates: 37.16 g

Starbucks® Pumpkin Scone

Preparation Time: 20 minutes

Cooking Time: 30 minutes

Servings: 6

Ingredients:

For Scones:

2 cups all-purpose flour

½ teaspoon each ground cinnamon & ground nutmeg

3 tablespoons half & half

1 tablespoon baking powder

¼ teaspoon each ground cloves & ground ginger

1 egg, large

6 tablespoons butter, cold

½ cup pumpkin, canned

7 tablespoons sugar

½ teaspoon salt

For Powdered Sugar Glaze:

2 tablespoons whole milk

1 cup plus 1 tablespoon powdered sugar

For Spiced Glaze

1 cup powdered sugar

3 tablespoons powdered sugar

2 tablespoons whole milk

¼ teaspoon ground cinnamon

1/8 teaspoon ground nutmeg

1 pinch of each ginger & ground cloves

Directions:

To Prepare the Scones:

Lightly oil a large sized baking sheet lined with a parchment paper & preheat your oven to 425 F.

Now, in a large sized bowl; combine flour together with baking powder, spices, salt & sugar; mix well. Cut the butter into the dry ingredients using a fork, pastry knife, or a food processor, until no obvious chunks of the butter & the mixture is crumbly; set aside.

Whisk pumpkin together with egg & half and half in a separate medium sized bowl. Mix wet ingredients with the dry ingredients; fold well & shape the dough into a ball.

Pat the dough out onto a lightly floured surface & make a 1" thick rectangle (approximately 3 inches wide & 9 inches long). Make three equal portions from the dough by slicing it twice through the width, using a pizza cutter or a large knife. Cut the slices diagonally until you get 6 triangular slices of the dough. Place them onto already prepared baking sheet & bake until turn lightly brown, for 12 to 15 minutes. Place them on a wire rack and let completely cool.

For the Plain Glaze:

Mix 2 tablespoon of milk together with the powdered sugar; mix well until completely smooth.

When you can handle the scones easily, paint the plain glaze on top of each scone using a brush.

For the Spiced Icing:

Combine the entire spicing ingredient together & drizzle this thicker icing on top of each scone; leave the icing for an hour and let dry, before serving. Drizzle with a whisk using a squirt bottle.

Nutrition: Calories: 507 kcal, Protein: 8.02 g, Fat: 17.69 g, Carbohydrates: 80.83 g

Starbucks® Coffee Cake

Preparation Time: 15 minutes

Cooking Time: 1 hour & 15 minutes

Servings: 8

Ingredients:

For the Batter

2 cups all-purpose flour

½ cup granulated sugar

2 eggs, large

1 cup softened butter

¾ cup packed sugar, light brown

1 ½ teaspoons vanilla

1/3 cup half & half

1 teaspoon of baking powder

¼ teaspoon salt

For Topping:

1 cup packed sugar, light brown

½ cup chopped pecans

1 cup all-purpose flour

½ cup softened butter

1 teaspoon cinnamon

Directions:

Preheat your oven to 325 F.

In a medium sized bowl; combine a cup of the flour with a stick of softened butter, brown sugar & 1 teaspoon of the cinnamon; mix well the mixture looks like moist sand. Add in half cup of pecans.

Now, using an electric mixer; cream 1 cup of butter together with ½ cup of granulated sugar & ¾ cup of light brown sugar until smooth & fluffy, in a large sized bowl. Add vanilla & eggs; mix well.

Combine flour together with baking powder & salt in a separate bowl. Combine the dry mixture with moist ingredients a small quantity at a time & then add in half & half; mix well.

Spoon the batter into a baking pan (9x13") lightly buttered & dusted with coating of flour.

Sprinkle the crumb topping on top of the batter. Ensure that the topping covers the batter completely.

Bake until the edges start to turn light brown, for 50 minutes. Let cool at room temperature & then slice into pieces.

Nutrition: Calories: 650 kcal, Protein: 6.71 g, Fat: 40.7 g, Carbohydrates: 66.09 g

Starbucks® Pumpkin Spice Latte

Preparation Time: 15 minutes

Cooking Time: 10 minutes

Servings: 1

Ingredients:

1 teaspoon vanilla simple syrup

1 cup coffee or 2 espresso shots

1 tablespoon pumpkin spice syrup

1 cup milk

For Garnish:

Whipped cream

Equal parts of pumpkin spice (ginger, cinnamon, ground clove, and nutmeg)

Directions:

Add milk together with vanilla syrup & pumpkin spice syrup into a microwave safe jar attached with a lid or a mason jar. Seal & shake until the milk is double in volume & frothy. Remove the lid & microwave until the milk is steamed, for a minute or two.

Transfer the hot milk either into coffee or espresso & top it first with the whipped cream & then a pinch of pumpkin spice.

Nutrition: Calories: 210 kcal, Protein: 8.3 g, Fat: 9.13 g, Carbohydrates: 25 g

Starbucks® Cranberry Bliss Bars

Preparation Time: 10 minutes

Cooking Time: 2 hours & 35 minutes

Servings: 40

Ingredients:

For Bars:

¾ cup white chocolate chips

2 sticks very soft butter (1 cup)

¾ cup dried cranberries (craisins)

3 eggs, large

2/3 cup to 1 cup brown sugar

2 cups all-purpose flour

⅓ cup granulated sugar

2 teaspoons vanilla or orange extract

1 ½ teaspoons baking powder

1 teaspoon ground ginger

For Topping:

½ teaspoon canola oil

1/3 cup white chocolate chips

1 -2 tablespoon orange rind, grated

1/3 cup chopped Craisins

For Frosting:

3 cups confectioners' sugar

1 teaspoon vanilla or orange extract

3 ounces softened cream cheese

2 tablespoons softened butter

Directions:

Line in a 10x15" pan with the parchment paper & preheat your oven to 350 F.

Beat softened butter together with sugars using an electric mixer, until light, for 3 to 5 minutes; gently blend in the orange extract and eggs (don't overbeat the eggs). Add in the flour, ginger & baking powder; beat for a short time. Add in the chips & cranberries, keep stirring until just incorporated.

Spread the batter into the already prepared pan & bake until the edges turn light brown, for 20 to 22 minutes. Don't over bake the bars or else they would become dry. Let them completely cool.

Now, blend butter & cream cheese until fluffy. Add confectioners' sugar & orange extract; beat until frosting is fluffy & spreadable (if required, feel free to add 1 teaspoon of milk). Spread it evenly over the cooled bars.

Remove the rind from an orange using a zester; sprinkle the zest on top of the frosted bars. Coarsely chop approximately 1/3 cup of the Craisins & then sprinkle on top of the frosted bars.

Now, in a glass measuring cup; mix oil & white chocolate. Microwave for a minute until melted; stirring after every 15 seconds. Whisk or use a fork to drizzle the melted white chocolate across the bars.

Before slicing into pieces, let it rest for an hour and let the white chocolate to completely set.

Nutrition: Calories: 156 kcal, Protein: 1.58 g, Fat: 7.4 g, Carbohydrates: 21.24 g

Soups and Side Dishes

Copycat Olive Garden's Creamy Zuppa Toscana

Preparation Time: 15 minutes

Cooking Time: 50 minutes

Servings: 4

Ingredients:

2 cups sweet yellow onion, quartered and sliced

½ cup sweet cream butter

½ teaspoon salt

1 tablespoon flour

4 cups beef stock

1 tablespoon fresh thyme

1 teaspoon coarse ground black pepper

4 baguette slices, approximately ½-inch thick

8 slices Provolone cheese

Directions:

Melt the butter in a stock pot over medium heat.

Add the onions and salt, and sauté for 3 minutes or until translucent but not browned. Add the flour and stir.

Add the beef stock, increase the heat to medium-high, and bring to a boil. Let boil for 1 minute.

Reduce the heat to low, season with thyme and black pepper. Cover and let simmer for 25-30 minutes.

While the soup is simmering, toast the baguette slices to a medium golden brown. Make sure each slice will fit comfortably in your soup bowl.

Preheat the broiler.

When the soup is done simmering, ladle it into oven proof serving bowls.

Top each bowl with a toasted baguette slice and 2 slices of Provolone cheese. Place under the broiler for 1-2 minutes, or until the cheese is well melted and lightly caramelized.

Remove from the broiler carefully and serve immediately

Nutrition: Calories: 420, Fat: 29 g, Carbs: 21 g, Protein: 19 g, Sodium: 2120 mg

Red Lobster's Clam Chowder

Preparation Time: 20 minutes

Cooking Time: 30 minutes

Servings: 8

Ingredients:

2 tablespoons butter

1 cup onion, diced

½ cup leek, white part, thinly sliced

¼ teaspoon garlic, minced

½ cup celery, diced

2 tablespoons flour

4 cups milk

1 cup clams with juice, diced

1 cup potato, diced

1 tablespoon salt

¼ teaspoon white pepper

1 teaspoon dried thyme

½ cup heavy cream

Saltine crackers for serving

Directions:

In a pot, sauté the onion, leek, garlic, and celery in butter over medium heat.

After 3 minutes, remove the vegetables from the heat and add the flour.

Whisk in the milk and clam juice.

Return the mixture to the heat and bring it to a boil.

Add the potatoes, salt, pepper, and thyme, then lower the heat to let the mixture simmer. Continue mixing for another 10 minutes while the soup is simmering.

Add in the clams and let the mixture simmer for 5 to 8 minutes, or until the clams are cooked.

Add the heavy cream and cook for a few more minutes.

Transfer the soup to a bowl and serve with saltine crackers.

Nutrition: Calories: 436.1, Fat: 26.5 g, Carbs: 30.1 g, Protein: 20.3 g, Sodium: 1987 mg

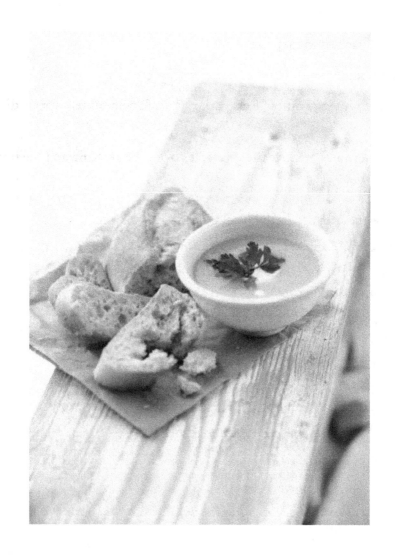

Carrabba's Mama Mandola Sicilian Chicken Soup

Preparation Time: 15 minutes

Cooking Time: 8 hours

Servings: 10

Ingredients:

4 carrots, peeled, diced

4 stalks celery, diced

1 green bell pepper, cored, diced

2 medium white potatoes, diced

1 white onion, diced

3 cloves garlic, minced

1 can (14.5 ounces) tomatoes, diced, with juice

1 tablespoon fresh parsley

1 teaspoon Italian seasoning

½ teaspoon white pepper

Dash of crushed red pepper flakes, to taste

2 boneless skinless chicken breasts, shredded

2 32-ounces containers chicken stock

1 ½ teaspoons salt

1 pound Ditalini pasta

Directions:

Dice and chop the vegetables as instructed.

Place them in a slow cooker and sprinkle with the parsley, seasoning, and white and red pepper. Mix everything together.

Add the shredded chicken and stock and mix again.

Cover the mixture and cook it for 8 hours on low heat.

When the soup is almost ready, bring a salt-and-water mixture to a boil to cook the pasta.

Add the cooked pasta to the soup and continue cooking for 5 minutes and serve.

Nutrition: Calories: 320, Fat: 0 g, Carbs: 57 g, Protein: 13 g, Sodium: 525.3 mg

Denny's Vegetable and Beef Barley Soup

Preparation Time: 10 minutes

Cooking Time: 40 minutes

Servings: 4

Ingredients:

½ pound ground beef

16 ounces frozen mixed vegetables

1 can (14.5 ounces) tomatoes, diced, with juice

¼ cup barley

32-ounce beef broth

Salt and pepper

Directions:

Place the ground beef in a pot and cook until brown.

Add in the vegetables, tomatoes, barley, and broth, and bring the entire mixture to a simmer.

Add salt and pepper for seasoning and leave the mixture to simmer for at least 40 minutes.

Ladle the soup into bowls and serve. The longer you leave the soup to simmer, the better it will taste.

Nutrition: Calories: 244.5, Fat: 11.4 g, Carbs: 17.1 g, Protein: 20 g, Sodium: 1818.2 mg

Outback's Walkabout Soup

Preparation Time: 10 minutes

Cooking Time: 45 minutes

Servings: 4

Ingredients:

Thick white Sauce:

3 tablespoons butter

3 tablespoons flour

¼ teaspoon salt

1½ cups whole milk

Soup:

2 cups yellow sweet onions, thinly sliced

3 tablespoons butter

1 can (14.5 ounces) chicken broth

½ teaspoon salt

¼ teaspoon fresh ground black pepper

2 chicken bouillon cubes

¼ cup Velveeta cubes, diced, packed

1½–1¾ cups white sauce (recipe above)

Cheddar cheese for garnish, shredded

Crusty bread for serving

Directions:

Make the thick white sauce first. Make a roux by cooking melted butter and flour over medium heat. Slowly pour the milk onto the roux, a little at a time, while constantly stirring the mixture. When the mixture reaches a pudding-like consistency, remove it from heat and set aside.

In a soup pot, sauté the onions in the butter over medium heat until they become translucent.

Add the rest of the ingredients, except the cheese and white sauce, to the pot and mix everything together.

When the mixture has heated up completely, add the cheese and white sauce. Bring the entire mixture to a simmer on medium-low heat. Continuously stir the soup until everything is completely mixed together.

When the cheese has melted, turn the heat lower and continue to cook the soup for another 30 to 45 minutes.

Ladle the soup into bowls and garnish with cheese. Serve with a side of bread.

Nutrition: Calories: 329, Fat: 25 g, Carbs: 17 g, Protein: 6 g, Sodium: 1061 mg

Wolfgang Puck's Butternut Squash Soup

Preparation Time: 25 minutes

Cooking Time: 1 hour and 15 minutes

Servings: 2 quarts

Ingredients:

Soup:

3¾ pounds butternut squash

1¾ pounds acorn squash

6 tablespoons unsalted butter, divided

1 onion, finely diced

½ teaspoon kosher salt

⅛ teaspoon fresh white pepper

¼ teaspoon ground nutmeg

¼ teaspoon ginger, ground

⅛ teaspoon ground cardamom

4 cups chicken or vegetable stock, warmed

½ cup crème fraiche

1 tablespoon thinly sliced fresh chives

Roasted Red Pepper Coulis:

2 red bell peppers

¼ cup chicken broth

Salt and pepper

Directions:

Preheat the oven to 350°F. Melt 2 tablespoons of the butter and season with salt, pepper, and nutmeg.

Prepare the squashes by cutting them in half, removing the seeds, and brushing the cut sides with the seasoned butter.

Line the squashes, cut-side down, on a baking pan. Bake for an hour.

When the squashes are soft, scoop them out into a bowl and purée. Set the squash purée aside.

Sauté the onions in 4 tablespoons of butter over low heat. Do not let them turn brown.

When the onions become translucent, add in the squash purée and allow the mixture to continue cooking. Make sure that the mixture does not simmer or boil.

When the mixture is heated through, add in the ginger and cardamom, then pour in the stock.

Without increasing the heat, bring the mixture to a boil. Allow the mixture to cook for 20 minutes while stirring occasionally.

Meanwhile, make the red pepper coulis:

a)   Roast the bell peppers over flame until the skin is charred or in oven under the broiler. Let the pepper cool down.

b)   Peel of the skin of the peppers and then purée the flesh while slowly pouring in the chicken broth.

c)   Season with salt and pepper.

d)   Transfer to a sauce bottle and set aside.

When the mixture has cooked through, add in the crème fraiche and chives.

When the flavors have mixed, remove the rosemary sprig and season the soup to your liking.

Transfer the mixture to a bowl and squeeze the red pepper coulis over the soup, creating swirls before serving.

Nutrition: Calories: 1293.8, Fat: 64.3 g, Carbs: 172.8 g, Protein: 27.9 g, Sodium: 1296.3 mg

Frijoles Negros (Cuban Black Beans)

Preparation Time: 30 minutes

Cooking Time: 1 hour

Servings: 8

Ingredients:

450 grams of black beans

10 cups of Water (2400 milliliters)

6 tablespoons olive oil

1 unit large onion

5 cloves of garlic

¼ tablespoon oregano dessert

1 bay leaf

¼ tablespoon ground cumin dessert

1 pinch of salt

1 pinch of pepper

1 tablespoon vinegar

1 tablespoon dry wine

1 tablespoon of sugar

1 unit large green chili pepper

Directions:

To start with our recipe for Cuban beans, the first thing we are going to do is to wash the beans well and soak them with water and a bay leaf. Ideally, leave them overnight so that they inflate and you can cook them better.

The next day, take a pot with enough capacity, pour the beans in it with the water and the bay leaf and cook them for approximately 45 minutes, until they are soft.

When they are ready, drain them and prepare the black bean stir - fry. To do this, take a deep pan and heat the olive oil. Once hot, add the finely chopped onion and chili, or crushed if desired, and crushed garlic. Remove it with a wooden spoon and fry it.

Of the already soft beans, reserve a cup for later, the rest add it to the frypan, with the blade included. Remove everything, add salt and pepper to taste, oregano, cumin, and sugar and simmer for a few minutes. Do not stop stirring to prevent black beans from sticking and burning.

Then, mash the beans you reserved in the cup, add them to the rest and simmer them for half an hour and with the pan covered.

After the time, add the dry wine and the vinegar, stir it well and let it rest with the fire for at least 10 minutes. When they are ready to add two tablespoons of olive oil, integrate it and serve the black beans to the Cuban accompanied by white rice.

Nutrition: Calories: 172kcal, Carbohydrates: 18 g, Fat: 9 g, Saturated fat: 5 g, Potassium: 369 mg, Protein: 6 g, Sodium: 294 mg, Fiber: 7 g, Sugar: 1 g, Vitamin A: 111IU, Vitamin C: 9 mg, Calcium: 23 mg, Iron: 1 mg

Oven Roasted Brussel Sprouts

Preparation Time: 50 minutes

Cooking Time: 30 minutes

Servings: 6

Ingredients:

500 grams of Brussels sprouts

3 tablespoons olive oil

2 tablespoons balsamic vinegar of Modena

2 tablespoons honey (or agave syrup or another sugar-free substitute)

Salt to taste Ground black pepper to taste

Directions:

Wash the cabbages and remove the top layers when necessary. We split them in half. Place the cabbage in a bowl and add the olive oil. We mix well.

Then, add the vinegar, honey or syrup and season to taste. We mix well.

Place the mixture on a baking sheet lined with vegetable paper with the inside of the cabbages facing up, and cook the Brussels sprouts in the oven and hot at 200°C at half-height about 20 minutes until golden brown and tender.

You will see how rich the roasted Brussels sprouts are left with that bittersweet mixture and the golden-brown of the oven. I can't think of a better way to enjoy this vegetable. Really, superior!

Nutrition: Calories: 357kcal, Carbohydrates: 42 g, Fat: 21 g, Saturated fat: 12 g, Carbs: 31 g, Protein: 5 g, Sodium: 334 mg, Sugar: 31 g, Fiber: 3 g, Vitamin A: 4598IU, Potassium: 503 mg, Vitamin C: 97 mg, Calcium: 116 mg, Iron: 2 mg

Garlic Green Beans

Preparation Time: 20 minutes

Cooking Time: 30 minutes

Servings: 10

Ingredients:

800 g of fresh green beans

2 cloves of garlic

1 tablet of vegetable broth

1 teaspoon chopped thyme

1 lemon

2 tablespoons olive oil

Salt

Directions:

Cut the ends of the beans, remove the strands and chop them. Peel and crush the garlic cloves together with the thyme in a mortar.

Put the oil in a pan and sauté the beans 3 or 4 minutes, add the mashed garlic and saute 3 more minutes over low heat, without letting the garlic burn.

Add water just to cover, pour the crumbled broth and salt to taste. Cook until the beans are tender (about 15-20 minutes), drain them and water them with the lemon juice.

Nutrition: Calories: 175kcal, Carbohydrates: 17 g, Saturated fat: 7 g, Cholesterol: 30 mg, Potassium: 479 mg, Fat: 12 g, Sugar: 7 g, Fiber: 6 g, Protein: 4 g, Sodium: 114 mg, Vitamin A: 1915IU, Vitamin C: 29 mg, Calcium: 89 mg, Iron: 2 mg

Souces and Dressing

Kraft Thousand Island dressing

Preparation Time: 5 minutes

Cooking Time: none

Servings: 16

Ingredients:

1 cup mayonnaise

¼ cup ketchup

2 tablespoons white vinegar

4 teaspoons white sugar

2 teaspoons sweet pickle relish, minced

2 teaspoons white onion, finely chopped or minced

¼ teaspoon sea salt

¼ teaspoon black pepper

Directions:

Take a large bowl and combine all the ingredients in it.

Mix well.

Serve.

Enjoy.

Nutrition: Calories: 67, Fat: 4.9 g, Carbs: 6 g, Protein: 2 g, Sodium: 167 mg

Newman Own's Creamy Caesar Salad Dressing

Preparation Time: 5 minutes

Cooking Time: 0

Servings: 10

Ingredients:

2 cups mayonnaise

6 tablespoons white vinegar, distilled

¼ cup Parmesan cheese, grated

4 teaspoons Worcestershire sauce

1 teaspoon lime juice

1 teaspoon dry mustard, ground   ⅓ teaspoon salt, or to taste

½ teaspoon garlic powder   ½ teaspoon onion powder

½ teaspoon black pepper, freshly ground

1 pinch basil, dried

1 pinch oregano, dried

Directions:

Take an electric mixer and blend all the ingredients until smooth.

Chill the prepared dressing for a few hours before severing.

Enjoy.

Nutrition: Calories: 215, Fat: 17.4 g, Carbs: 13.3 g, Protein: 2.3 g, Sodium: 540 mg

Bull's Eye Original BBQ Sauce

Preparation Time: 20 minutes

Cooking Time: 15 minutes

Servings: yield 2 cups

Ingredients:

1½ cups tomato ketchup

½ cup Worcestershire sauce

5 tablespoons butter, melted

¼ cup white vinegar

1 tablespoon yellow mustard

¼ cup onions, finely minced

2 tablespoons hickory liquid smoke

½ teaspoon Tabasco sauce

1 cup sugar, brown

1 tablespoon white sugar

Salt, to taste

Directions:

Combine the ingredients in a saucepan and heat it over medium heat.

Simmer the ingredients for 15 minutes, stirring occasionally.

Turn off the heat and let the sauce get cold.

The sauce is ready.

Nutrition: Calories: 112, Fat: 3.7 g, Carbs: 20.5 g, Protein: 0.5 g, Sodium: 386 mg

Kraft Miracle Whip

Preparation Time: 20 minutes

Cooking Time: 15 minutes

Servings: 1 ½ cups

Ingredients:

4 egg yolks

⅓ teaspoon salt

2 tablespoons powdered sugar

6 tablespoons lemon juice

2 cups oil

2 tablespoons cornstarch

2 teaspoons dry mustard

1 cup boiling water

¼ cup vinegar

Table salt, to taste

Directions:

Take a blender and add egg yolks along with salt, sugar, and half of lemon juice.

Blend for few seconds until combined.

While the blender is running, start adding the oil, a few drops at a time.

Add the remaining lemon juice.

Turn off the blender.

In a bowl, mix together cornstarch, water, mustard, and vinegar.

Mix until a smooth paste is formed.

Pour the bowl ingredients into a pan.

Cook on low heat until thickened.

Slowly add this cooked mixture into the blender.

Turn on the blender and combine all the ingredients well.

Transfer to a jar and let cool in the refrigerator.

Nutrition: Calories: 432, Fat: 49. 1g, Carbs: 0. 9 g, Protein: 4.3 g, Sodium: 564 mg

Hellman's Mayonnaise

Preparation Time: 15 minutes

Cooking Time: none

Servings: 1 cup

Ingredients:

3 large egg yolks

1 teaspoon dry mustard

1 teaspoon salt

½ teaspoon cayenne pepper

1½ cups canola oil

4-6 tablespoons lemon juice

Directions:

Add mustard and egg yolks into a blender and pulse until combined.

While the blender is blending set the speed to low and start adding the oil very slowly.

Stop the blender and scrape down the mayonnaise.

Add the lemon juice and remaining oil.

Keep on blending until combined.

At the end add salt and cayenne pepper.

Mix and serve.

Nutrition: Calories: 362, Fat: 39.1, Carbs: 0.7 g, Protein: 3.4 g, Sodium: 425 mg

Heinz Ketchup

Preparation Time: 25 minutes

Cooking Time: 20 minutes

Servings: yield about 1 and ½ cups

Ingredients:

1 cup tomato paste

⅓ cup light corn syrup

½ cup white vinegar

⅓ cup water

2 tablespoons sugar

Salt, to taste

⅓ teaspoon onion powder

¼ teaspoon garlic powder

Directions:

Combine all the ingredients in a saucepan.

Turn on the heat and let the liquid simmer for 20 minutes.

Turn off the heat and let the mixture cool down.

Store in airtight glass jar or serve with French fries.

Nutrition: Calories: 78, Fat: 0.2 g, Carbs: 19.3 g, Protein: 1.4 g, Sodium: 53 mg

Hidden Valley Original Ranch Dressing

Preparation Time: 10 minutes

Cooking Time: none

Servings: 6

Ingredients:

1 cup mayonnaise

1 cup buttermilk

1 teaspoon parsley flakes, dried

½ teaspoon black pepper, ground

⅓ teaspoon sea salt

¼ teaspoon garlic powder

¼ teaspoon onion powder

2 pinches of thyme, dried

Directions:

Take a blender and combine all the ingredients in it.

Pulse until smooth.

Transfer to a glass jar and chill in refrigerator before serving.

Nutrition: Calories: 170, Fat: 13.5 g, Carbs: 11.7 g, Protein: 1.8 g, Sodium: 427 mg

Carrabba's Bread Dipping Blend

Preparation Time: 10 minutes

Cooking Time: 10 minutes

Servings: 8

Ingredients:

1 tablespoon red pepper, crushed

1 ½ teaspoon garlic powder

1 tablespoon dried parsley

½ teaspoon dried rosemary

1 tablespoon dried basil

1 ½ teaspoon onion powder

1 tablespoon dried oregano

3 garlic cloves, fresh, crushed

Extra virgin olive oil, as required

1 tablespoon freshly cracked black pepper

1 ½ teaspoon coarse sea salt

Directions:

Combine black pepper together with the parsley, crushed red pepper, basil, oregano, onion powder, garlic powder, rosemary, crush garlic and sea salt; mix well.

Place the dry spice mixture in a large-sized shallow plate & drizzle with the extra virgin olive oil. Mix well & serve.

Nutrition: Calories: 243, Fat: 89.3 g, Carbs: 15.4 g, Protein: 24.8 g, Sodium: 1687 mg

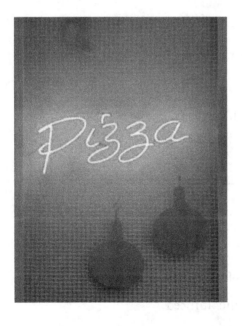

California Pizza Kitchen Tuscan Hummus

Preparation Time: 30 minutes

Cooking Time: 30 minutes

Servings: 6

Ingredients:

10 garlic cloves

½ cup tahini or sesame paste

2 cans great northern or cannellini beans, drained (15-ounce size)

1/8 teaspoon ground coriander

1 tablespoon plus ½ teaspoon soy sauce

¼ cup lemon juice, freshly squeezed

1 ½ teaspoon cumin

½ teaspoon cayenne pepper

2 tablespoons fresh Italian parsley, minced

1 ½ teaspoon salt

¼ cup cold water, if required

For California Pizza Kitchen Checca:

2 pounds Roma tomatoes, cut into ½" dice

1 tablespoon fresh basil, minced

½ cup extra-virgin olive oil

1 tablespoon garlic, minced

2 teaspoons salt

Directions:

Process the garlic cloves in a food processor attached with a steel blade until minced finely, stopping & scrapping the sides of the work bowl occasionally, as required.

Add in the cannellini beans & pulse again until coarsely chopped. Then, with the machine still running on low speed, slowly pour the sesame paste through the feed tube & puree. Don't just turn off the motor; pour in the soy sauce, olive oil and lemon juice through the feed tube (stopping & scrapping down the sides, as required).

Stop; remove the lid & add cumin, cayenne, coriander and salt. Process again until blended thoroughly. Feel free to add ¼ to ½ cup of cold water to the mix and pulse, if the puree seems to be too thick for spreading or dipping. Transfer the puree to a large bowl & cover with a plastic wrap; let refrigerate until chill.

In the meantime; preheat your oven to 250 F in advance.

Place the pita breads in the preheated oven & heat for a couple of minutes, until thoroughly warmed.

Carefully remove the breads & cut into desired wedges. Place the chilled hummus in a serving bowl or plate & arrange the tomato Checca over the top. Garnish with the freshly chopped parsley & surround with the pita triangles. Serve immediately and enjoy.

For California Pizza Kitchen Checca:

Toss the entire Checca ingredients together in a large-sized mixing bowl; continue to toss until thoroughly mixed. Using a plastic wrap; cover & refrigerate until ready to use.

Nutrition: Calories: 134, Fat: 67 g, Carbs: 52. 5 g, Protein: 64 g, Sodium: 1254 mg

Cheddar's Santa Fe Spinach Dip

Preparation Time: 5 minutes

Cooking Time: 20 minutes

Servings: 6

Ingredients:

2 packages chopped spinach, frozen (10 ounces each)

1 cup heavy whipping cream

2.4 ounces Monterey jack cheese; cut it into 3 equal 2" long blocks

1 package cream cheese (8 oz)

2.4 ounces pepper jack cheese; cut it into 3 equal 2" long blocks

½ cup Sour Cream

2.4 ounces White American Cheese; cut it into 3 equal 2" long blocks

½ to 1 teaspoon salsa seasoning

2 teaspoon Alfredo sauce

1 cup mozzarella cheese

Pepper & salt to taste

Directions:

Over low-heat in a large pan; heat the chopped spinach until all the moisture is cooked out, for a couple of minutes, stirring frequently.

In the meantime, over moderate heat in a large pot; add in the cream cheese & 1 cup of heavy whipping cream; cook until the cheese is completely melted; ensure that you don't really bring it to a boil. Feel free to decrease the heat, if it starts to boil.

Once done; work in batches and start adding the Pepper Jack, Monterey Jack & White American cheeses. Continue to stir the ingredients & don't let it come to a boil.

Lastly add in the Mozzarella cheese and continue to cook.

Add 2 teaspoons of the Alfredo sauce and then add in the cooked spinach.

Add ½ cup of the sour cream; continue to mix until combined well.

Add salsa seasoning, pepper & salt to taste; stir well

Serve immediately with some tortilla chips & enjoy!

Nutrition: Calories: 177, Fat: 12. 6 g, Carbs: 35. 8 g, Protein: 37. 8 g, Sodium: 677 mg

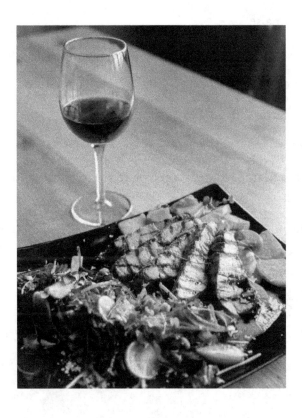

Olive Garden Hot Artichoke Spinach Dip

Preparation Time: 30 minutes

Cooking Time: 30 minutes

Servings: 4

Ingredients:

½ cup chopped spinach, frozen, thawed & well drained

1 package (8-ounce size) cream cheese, at room temperature

¼ cup each of Mozzarella cheese, Romano cheese & Parmesan cheese, shredded

1 garlic clove, minced finely

¼ cup mayonnaise

1 can artichoke hearts, drained & coarsely chopped (14 ounce)

½ teaspoon dried basil

¼ teaspoon garlic salt

Directions:

Lightly grease a large-sized glass pie plate and preheat your oven to 350 F in advance.

Beat the cream cheese together with Romano cheese, Parmesan cheese, mayonnaise, basil, garlic & garlic salt in a large-sized mixing bowl; beat well.

Stir in the spinach and artichoke hearts until mixed well.

When ready, spoon the dip into the greased pie plate & evenly sprinkle the top with the Mozzarella cheese.

Place the dip in the oven and bake until the Mozzarella cheese is completely melted & turns lightly browned, for 25 minutes, at 350 F.

Remove the dip from oven & serve hot with some crackers or toasted bread slices for dipping.

Nutrition: Calories: 143, Fat: 6.9 g, Carbs: 65 g, Protein: 26 g, Sodium: 376 mg

Olive Garden Spinach-Artichoke Dip

Preparation Time: 3 minutes

Cooking Time: 35 minutes

Servings: 10

Ingredients:

1 can artichoke hearts, drained, coarsely chopped (14 ounce)

¼ cup mayonnaise

1 package light cream cheese (8 ounce); at room temperature

¼ cup parmesan cheese

½ cup chopped spinach, frozen

¼ cup Romano cheese

1 garlic clove, minced finely

¼ cup mozzarella cheese, grated

½ teaspoon dry basil or 1 tablespoon fresh

¼ teaspoon garlic salt

Pepper & salt to taste

Directions:

Combine cream cheese together with mayonnaise Romano cheese, Parmesan, basil, garlic & garlic salt; mix until combined well.

Add in the drained spinach and artichoke hearts; mix until well blended.

Spray a pie pan with Pam and then pour in the dip; top with the Mozzarella cheese.

Bake until the top is browned, for 25 minutes, at 350 F.

Serve with Italian or French toasted bread, thinly sliced.

Nutrition: Calories: 563, Fat: 14. 3 g, Carbs: 76. 8 g, Protein: 54. 8 g, Sodium: 1434. 7 mg

Houston's Chicago Style Spinach Dip

Preparation Time: 5 minutes

Cooking Time: 15 minutes

Servings: 10

Ingredients:

⅓ cup sour cream

2 bags of fresh Spinach (1 pound each)

⅔ cup fresh parmesan cheese, grated

1 can Artichoke Hearts, coarsely diced

1/8 pound butter

2 tablespoons onions, minced

½ cup Monterrey Jack Cheese, grated

1 teaspoon fresh garlic, minced

½ teaspoon Tabasco sauce or to taste

1 pint heavy whipping cream

¼ cup flour

2 teaspoons lemon juice, freshly squeezed

½ teaspoon salt

Directions:

Steam the spinach; strain & using a cheese cloth; squeeze the water out. Finely chop & set aside until ready to use.

Now, over moderate heat in a heavy saucepan; heat the butter until completely melted.

Add in the onions and garlic; sauté for 3 to 5 minutes.

Make a roux by adding the flour. Give everything a good stir & cook for a minute.

Slowly add in the heavy cream, stirring with a whisk to prevent lumping. The mixture would thicken at the boiling point.

When done, immediately add in the Tabasco, lemon juice, Parmesan cheese and salt.

Immediately remove the pan from heat & let stand at room temperature for 5 minutes and then stir in the sour cream.

Fold in the diced artichoke hearts, Jack cheese and dry & chopped spinach. Stir well until the cheese is completely melted.

Serve immediately and enjoy.

Nutrition: Calories: 476. 6, Fat: 53. 6 g, Carbs: 78. 7 g, Protein: 27. 7 g, Sodium: 2868 mg

Ruby Tuesday Queso Dip

Preparation Time: 10 minutes

Cooking Time: 10 minutes

Servings: 6

Ingredients:

1 box chopped spinach, frozen, thawed & squeeze out any excess water (approximately 10 oz)

1 jar of Taco Bell salsa & queso (approximately 14 oz)

Directions:

Mix the entire ingredients together in a microwave-safe bowl. Heat in 1-minute intervals on high-power, stirring frequently. Continue to heat in the microwave until heated through. Serve with your favorite tortilla chips and enjoy.

Nutrition: Calories: 257, Fat: 47.7 g, Carbs: 86. 6 g, Protein: 28. 7 g, Sodium: 2498 mg

Desserts

Panera Bread's Chocolate Chip Cookies

Preparation Time: 15 minutes

Cooking Time: 15 minutes

Servings: 12

Ingredients:

2½ sticks unsalted butter

1¼ cup dark brown sugar

¼ cup granulated sugar

2 teaspoons vanilla extract

2 eggs

3½ cups all-purpose flour

1 tablespoon cornstarch

1 teaspoon baking soda

1 teaspoon salt

1 bag (12 ounces) mini semisweet chocolate chips

Directions:

Cream the butter and sugars using a whisk or a hand mixer.

Whip in the vanilla extract and eggs and set the wet mixture aside.

In a different bowl, mix together the flour, cornstarch, baking soda, and salt.

Pour the dry mixture into the wet mixture a little at a time, folding with a spatula. Add in the chocolate chips and continue folding.

Roll the cookie dough into balls and place them on a baking sheet. Place the baking sheet in the freezer for 15 minutes.

Preheat the oven to 350°F while waiting for the cookies to harden.

Transfer the cookies from the freezer to the oven immediately and bake for 15 minutes.

Nutrition: Calories: 440, Fat: 23 g, Carbs: 59 g, Protein: 4 g, Sodium: 240 mg

Applebee's Maple Butter Blondie

Preparation Time: 10 minutes

Cooking Time: 25 minutes

Servings: 6

Ingredients:

⅓ cup butter, melted

1 cup brown sugar, packed

1 egg, beaten

1 tablespoon vanilla extract

1 cup all-purpose flour

½ teaspoon baking powder

⅛ teaspoon baking soda

⅛ teaspoon salt

½ cup white chocolate chips

½ cup walnuts or pecans, chopped

Maple Cream Sauce:

½ cup maple syrup

¼ cup butter

½ cup brown sugar

8 ounces cream cheese, softened

Walnuts for garnish, chopped; optional

Vanilla ice cream for serving

Directions:

Prepare your materials by:

a)   Preheating the oven to 350°F; and

b)   Greasing an 8×8 baking pan.

Dissolve the sugar in the melted butter. Whip in the egg and the vanilla and set the mixture aside.

In another bowl, mix together the flour, baking powder and soda, and salt.

Slowly pour the dry mixture into the butter mixture and mix thoroughly.

Make sure the mixture is at room temperature before folding in the nuts and chocolate chips.

Transfer the mixture into the baking pan and bake for 20 to 25 minutes.

While waiting for the blondies to bake, combine the syrup and butter over low heat. When the butter has melted, mix in the sugar and cream cheese. Take the mixture off the heat when the cream cheese has melted, and set aside.

Let the blondies cool a little and then cut them into rectangles. Serve with the syrup, top with walnuts and vanilla ice cream, if desired, and serve.

Nutrition: Calories: 1000, Fat: 54 g, Carbs: 117 g, Protein: 13 g, Sodium: 620 mg

Tommy Bahama's Key Lime Pie

Preparation Time: 40 minutes

Cooking Time: 50 minutes

Servings: 2

Ingredients:

Pie:

10-inch graham cracker crust

1 egg white

2½ cups sweetened condensed milk

¾ cup pasteurized egg yolk

1 cup lime juice

1 lime, zest

1 lime, sliced into 8

White Chocolate Mousse Whipped Cream:

8 fluid ounces heavy cream

3 tablespoons powdered sugar

¼ teaspoon pure vanilla extract

½ tablespoon white chocolate mousse instant mix

Directions:

Preheat the oven to 350°F while brushing the graham cracker crust with the egg white. Cover the crust completely before placing it in the oven to bake for 5 minutes.

Whip the egg yolk and condensed milk together until they are blended completely. Add the lime juice and zest to the mixture and continue whipping until the mixture is smooth.

If you haven't yet, remove the crust from the oven and let it cool. When the crust has cooled, add in the egg mixture and bake at 250°F for 25 to 30 minutes.

When the pie is cooked, place it on a cooling rack to cool. Then place it in the refrigerator for at least two hours.

While waiting for the pie to cool, beat the first three whipped cream ingredients for two minutes (if using a hand mixer). When the mixture is smooth, add in the chocolate mousse and beat to stiff peaks.

Remove the pie from the refrigerator, slice it into eight pieces, and garnish each with the white chocolate mousse whipped cream and a slice of lime. Serve.

Nutrition: Calories: 500, Fat: 9 g, Carbs: 26 g, Protein: 1 g, Sodium: 110 mg

Dairy Queen's Blizzard

Preparation Time: 5 minutes

Cooking Time: 0 minutes

Servings: 1

Ingredients:

1 candy bar, of your choice

¼ to ½ cup milk

2½ cups vanilla ice cream

1 teaspoon fudge sauce

Directions:

Place the candy bar of your choice into the freezer to harden it.

Break the candy bar into multiple tiny chunks and place all the ingredients into a blender.

Keep blending until the ice cream becomes thicker and everything is mixed completely.

Pour into a cup and consume.

Nutrition: Calories: 953, Fat: 51.6 g, Carbs: 108.8 g, Protein: 15.1 g, Sodium: 439.4 mg

Olive Garden's Tiramisu

Preparation Time: 10 minutes

Cooking Time: 2 hours and 50 minutes

Servings: 9

Ingredients:

4 egg yolks

2 tablespoons milk

⅔ cup granulated sugar

2 cups mascarpone cheese

¼ teaspoon vanilla extract

1 cup heavy cream

½ cup cold espresso

¼ cup Kahlua

20–24 ladyfingers

2 teaspoons cocoa powder

Directions:

Bring water to a boil, then reduce the heat to maintain a simmer. Place a heatproof bowl over the water, making sure that the bowl does not touch the water.

In the heatproof bowl, whisk together the egg yolks, milk and sugar for about 8 to 10 minutes.

When the mixture has thickened, remove the bowl from heat and then whisk in the vanilla and mascarpone cheese until the mixture becomes smooth.

In another bowl, whisk the cream until soft peaks are formed.

Using a spatula, fold the whipped cream into the mascarpone mixture, making sure to retain the fluffiness of the whipped cream.

In another bowl, mix the espresso and Kahlua.

Dip the ladyfingers into the espresso mixture one by one. Dip only the bottom, and dip them quickly so as not to make them soggy.

Cover the bottom of an 8×8 pan with half of the dipped ladyfingers, cracking them if necessary.

Pour half of the mascarpone mixture over the ladyfingers.

Place another layer of ladyfingers over the mixture.

Pour the rest of the mixture over the second layer of ladyfingers and smooth out the top.

Dust some cocoa powder over the top and then place in the refrigerator.

Slice the cake and serve when set.

Nutrition: Calories: 288.6, Fat: 14 g, Carbs: 34.4 g, Protein: 4.4 g, Sodium: 53.6 mg

Cheesecake Factory's Oreo Cheesecake

Preparation Time: 25 minutes

Cooking Time: 1 hour

Servings: 10

Ingredients:

Crust:

1½ cups Oreo cookies, crushed

2 tablespoons butter, melted

Filling:

3 packages (8 ounces each) cream cheese, room temperature

1 cup sugar

5 large eggs, room temperature

2 teaspoons vanilla extract

¼ teaspoon salt

¼ cup all-purpose flour

1 container (8 ounces) sour cream, room temperature

14 Oreo cookies, divided

Directions:

To make the crust, crush whole Oreos in a blender or smash them with a rolling pin and mix them with the melted butter. Press the Oreo mixture to the bottom and sides of a 9-inch spring form pan.

Leave the crust to rest and preheat the oven to 325°F. Before starting to make the filling, make sure all of your ingredients are at room temperature.

Place the cream cheese in a medium-sized bowl and beat it with a hand mixer or a whisk until it is light and fluffy.

Beat in the sugar, mixing continuously so that the sugar is evenly distributed throughout the mixture.

Beat in the eggs, one at a time, and then add in the vanilla, salt, and flour. When the ingredients are all mixed together, add in the sour cream and 6 chopped Oreos.

Pour the filling onto the crust and then top with 8 whole Oreos.

Bake in the oven for an hour to an hour and 15 minutes. When the cake is done baking, leave it in the oven with the door open for an hour.

When it has cooled down, transfer the cake to the refrigerator. Leave it for a day or more before serving.

Nutrition: Calories: 1520, Fat: 55 g, Carbs: 175 g, Protein: 0 g, Sodium: 736 mg

P.F. Chang's Ginger Panna Cotta

Preparation Time: 10 minutes

Cooking Time: 4 hours and 10 minutes

Servings: 3

Ingredients:

Panna Cotta:

¼ cup heavy cream

½ cup granulated sugar

1 tablespoon grated ginger

1½ tablespoons powdered gelatin

6 tablespoons warm water

Strawberry Sauce:

2 pounds ripe strawberries, hulled

½ cup granulated sugar

2 teaspoons cornstarch

½ lemon, juice

1 pinch salt

Directions:

Place the cream, sugar and ginger in a saucepan and cook over medium-low heat, until the sugar dissolves. Remove the mixture from heat and set aside.

In a medium-sized bowl, mix the water and the gelatin together. Set aside for a few minutes.

After the gelatin has rested, pour the sugar mixture into the medium-sized bowl and stir, removing all lumps.

Grease your ramekins and then transfer the mixture into the ramekins, leaving 2 inches of space at the top.

Place the ramekins in your refrigerator or freezer to let them set for at least 4 hours.

While the panna cottas are setting, make the strawberry sauce by cooking all the sauce ingredients in a medium-sized pan for 10 minutes. Stir the mixture occasionally, then remove from heat.

When the panna cottas are ready, flip over the containers onto a plate and allow the gelatin to stand. Drizzle with the strawberry sauce and serve.

Nutrition: Calories: 346, Fat: 30 g, Carbs: 16 g, Protein: 4 g, Sodium: 50 mg

Conclusion

When preparing desserts at home, you can tweak the recipes as you wish. As you sample the recipes, you'll get to know the usual ingredients and techniques in making popular sweet treats. This could inspire you to create your very own recipes. You can substitute ingredients as your taste, health or pocket dictates. You can come up, perhaps, not with a dessert that's the perfect clone of a restaurant's recipe, but with one that's exactly the way you want it to be. Most of all, the recipes here are meant for you to experience the fulfillment of seeing the smiles on the people with whom you share your creations. Keep trying and having fun with these recipes and you'll soon be reaping your sweet rewards!

Reasons Copycat Recipes Are Better Than Eating at Restaurants

Imagine sitting at your favorite restaurant in the booth and your waitress has just placed your favorite hot piping dish before you. Smells so sweet! But it can be very expensive to eat out several times a week. What if you could have the exact recipe to make your favorite dish whenever you wish? What if you had over 100 home-made restaurant recipes to fix? Do the copycat recipes taste the real thing?

We are doing that, totally! Copycat recipes are constantly being tested to ensure that you create the restaurant's exact dishes. Expert chefs spend hours tailoring these recipes to get the perfect flavor. Such recipes are as close to the real thing as being in your own kitchen right at your favorite restaurant. How will you save money on these copycat recipes?

With these recipes the amount of money you'll save will be absolutely shocking. Imagine spending a night out at your favorite restaurant, for you and your significant other. You get an appetizer, 2 begins and a dessert is shared. You spent between $55 and $70 comfortably with beverages, food and a tip. You will probably spend about a third of that on producing these same recipes at home without losing any taste. So you could use the copycat recipes to prepare 3 different meals at home for what it would cost you to eat out once. So where are these recipes you looking at?

That's the copycat recipe's great thing. You won't need any special cooking appliances or any special ingredients. If you do any cooking, you probably already have the things you need around your kitchen. Whatever you don't have should be readily available at your local food mart. There's nothing exotic about this.

Think back to the last time you've been to your favorite restaurant. Was there a line? When seated, how did you anxiously wait for your favorite meal to arrive? Then that feeling came when the waitress put it on the table. Finally, ahhh, was it perfect? Or was it not? Like it just wasn't cooked right. Or maybe it wasn't warm enough or they left a topping out? What did you feel when you got this bill? Did 'Aahhh' become 'woooah'? I'll show you how you can stop such problems associated with eating out. It's all by using reliable and proven copycat recipes. Want to know the top five reasons to make your favorite home-made foods?

Cost

How much do copycat recipes actually save you? Let's say you're out to eat with your significant other. Now let's add some drinks and a tip. You have invested $60-$80 comfortably anywhere in the neighborhood. You get an appetizer, two exits, and perhaps a dessert is split. You might have made the same meal at home for $25-$30, less than half the eating out price! And in the meantime, don't lose any flavor. That is a huge saving in these economic times. That sounds great but we are talking about how many recipes?

Health

That's the wonderful thing about making home copycat recipes. They give you the exact ingredients, but whatever you see fit, you can change them. Whether to give a different flavor to the food, or add your own homegrown vegetables. You can also add ingredients lower in fat, or remove ingredients to which you are allergic. The possibilities are endless. You are in full control of that. Like the original dishes, how do you learn how these recipes taste?

Quality

A team of professional chefs created these recipes. We have checked over and over to make sure you get the exact ingredients and correct steps to make your favorite dish. You can of course go online to find recipes which claim to be copycats of popular restaurants. Yes, it's free. And it's a reason they're free. These are not real recipes for copycat purposes. They are actually not even close. I've tried a couple and to be honest, they weren't close, they weren't even good. I'll show you how to get the real copycat recipes and get your freedom back.

Freedom

Will you know how much you waste eating out of your time and freedom? Can you get the midnight meal you prefer? When watching your favorite series, will you eat your favorite meal? For instance, you are driving to the restaurant, waiting to sit down, waiting to get your appetizer, waiting to get your meal, waiting to get your dessert and, you guessed it, waiting to pay your bill. So, how much you did wait? Two hours, three more hours? Take your time and freedom back, and fix your favorite meals at home. Use these copycat recipes when you want to make your favorite meal and how you want it.

All of these dishes are custom-tested and customer-approved restaurants. Do you have an enjoyable meal at a restaurant and would like to replicate it at home? There are a few cloned restaurant recipes now, because some of you have been asking for them. Almost every one of us went to a restaurant and had a meal that was so delicious that we wanted to know how to make that meal at home. There is a staggering increase in interest in discovering online restaurants.

Have you ever wondered what the "Chef's" secrets are that made all the restaurant's famous dishes? Real Restaurant Recipes, sauce and gravy dishes, are hidden recipes for a number of sauce restaurants; each is a popular home-made dish. There's a multitude of books out there that have unnecessary copycat dishes of the popular top-secret recipes. How can I learn to cook those popular dishes in the restaurant?

Cooking also shows that there is no shortcut to performance. You can substitute less healthy ingredients for healthier ingredients when you prepare those famous restaurant recipes at home. Now, I will create my own meals and present them whenever I cook. Getting into the habit of eating at home is a hard thing, but learning how to cook your favorite restaurant meals in the comfort of your own kitchen can make it a little easier. It's not really that hard to learn how to cook secret restaurant meals. People think you need a background in cooking or a degree in culinary arts to be able to cook those secret dishes. What better way to control the consistency of what you and your family shove into your mouth than by preparing your own meals? Today, this remains the best reason to learn to cook: because you can.

CPSIA information can be obtained
at www.ICGtesting.com
Printed in the USA
BVHW081410091120
592845BV00014B/1270